What *Diet Trials* participants had to say about their weight-loss experiences:

'The meetings help you plan and give you the drive to stay on the right track. I've had some hard days and some really bad days, but I will carry on and I will get into that bikini!' Gillian

'I'm enjoying my diet because it isn't too different from what I eat normally – just less of it and lower in fat.' Julia

'My diet is boring! But I do feel quite positive about my progress so far and I'm very confident about keeping the weight off long term.' Scott

'When the weight fell off over the first month, I loved the diet, but now my weight is at a standstill and I've lost heart in it. But I will stick it out – I'm determined!' Georgina

'My main reason for wanting to lose weight is to be healthier. I'm enjoying my diet but it is very restrictive.' Hector

'I am enjoying the diet because I am able to eat foods I like. I am a hundred per cent confident about keeping off the weight in the long term. I thought I was destined to be big all my life. I've wasted so many years with that stupid thought.' Linda

'The most useful aspect of my diet is retraining my attitude towards food. My biggest problem when it came to controlling my weight was lack of exercise.' Kerry

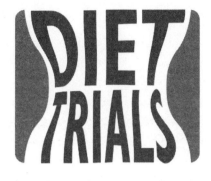

how to succeed at dieting

by Lyndel Costain BSc SRD

with a foreword by Eamonn Holmes

For Steve

This book is published to accompany the BBC series *Diet Trials* which was first broadcast in 2003. Editor: Lisa Ausden; Series Producer: Gaby Koppel.

A BBCi website offering advice and information is available at
www.bbc.co.uk/diettrials

Published by BBC Worldwide Limited, Woodlands, 80 Wood Lane, London W12 0TT
First published 2003

Text © Lyndel Costain 2003
Foreword © Eamonn Holmes 2003

The moral right of the authors has been asserted.

ISBN 0 563 48872 7

Commissioning Editor: Rachel Copus
Project Editor: Julia Charles
Copy Editor: Tessa Clarke
Design Manager: Sarah Ponder
Designer: Peter Coombs
Production controller: Kenneth McKay

Set in Foundry Sans
Printed and bound in Great Britain by Bath Press Ltd.
Cover printed by Belmont Press, Northampton

While the author has made every effort to provide accurate and up-to-date information, nutritional science is constantly evolving. You should always consult a doctor or dietitian for individualized health and medical advice.

Author acknowledgments: I would like to thank the many dietitians, nutrition scientists, doctors and associations who provided information to help make this book happen. Not to mention the many people I have been fortunate enough to work with to manage – and feel better about – their weight. Particular thanks go to: Dympna Pearson SRD, Trainer in Behaviour Change Skills; Dr Susan Jebb, Head of Nutrition and Health Research, Medical Research Council Human Nutrition Research, Cambridge; Dr David Ashton, Director of the UK Women's Heart Study and the Healthier Weight Clinic, Birmingham; The Association for the Study of Obesity.

contents

foreword

If there is one thing that a diet is it's certainly a trial! With this series of TV programmes though, we set out to put the diets on trial instead of you. There's no real need to ask why I am presenting the *Diet Trials*. I'd love to say it was because of my keen investigative brain but sadly one look at me says it all – I'm overweight. Not only that, but I'm a bit of a rarity. I'm an overweight TV presenter and there aren't many of those to a dozen!

So, like you, I had a go at dieting – bought the latest get-fit gizmos and gadgets and stuck at whatever the latest fad was until whatever brief weight loss it initially brought slowed up. That's me – no stamina, no staying power, no faith. No real faith in the claims diets make and as a result I suppose no real faith in myself or my ability to last the course. *Diet Trials* interested the sceptic in me. Which one would work and who would it work for? Was I always the problem or could it sometimes be the diet?

Diet Trials is not about jumping on to the latest 'celebrity diet' bandwagon, or starving yourself for two weeks to look fabulous for your holiday, in fact, that's exactly what both the television series and this book are trying to help you avoid.

If you're reading this book, the chances are that you are feeling in need of losing the odd pound or two. Well, let me reassure you, you're not alone. Over half the adults in this country are overweight, and one in five of us is at least two-to-three stone overweight. What's more, as a nation we're getting fatter, too. Of course, these are depressing statistics and it's very easy to shrug them off, only remembering them when we're faced with the brutal fact that we can't get into last year's clothes anymore. But it really is worth keeping them in mind, not just because by losing weight you'll look better, but because you'll feel better too and will have a longer and healthier life into the bargain.

The fact that so many of us are overweight leads naturally on to the fact that at any one time millions of us are dieting. Each year brings us a new kind of diet to try that seems to guarantee weight-loss success, and every year many of us give them a try (go on, admit it, I bet you've experimented with at least one of them). Armed with this knowledge, scientists from the University of Surrey got together with the BBC to conduct a unique project, the first scientific weight-loss experiment to research commercially available diets. *Diet Trials*, the series, is the result.

Focussed around four of Britain's best-known diets, the aim of the experiment was to discover which diet was the most effective, which diet was the most healthy for your body and which diet helped you to lose the most weight. Three hundred dieters were selected and allotted one of the diets at random. At the end of the six months the results will be collected together and the outcome announced on television.

I have to say that it's been absolutely fascinating to hear how the dieters are getting on. As time has gone by and we've got to know some of the dieters better, we've all really experienced the highs and lows of their weight-loss programme ... and learned an awful lot about the different diets, too. I can honestly say that at the time of writing this foreword we don't know what the results are going to be, but we're all waiting with bated breath to find out!

Hats off to the dieters, too. Over the six months that we've been filming *Diet Trials* I have grown to admire many of the participants. They have allowed themselves to be weighed and measured and photographed, and, of course, they have all made a commitment to trying to lose weight. By buying this book you have also made that commitment, so well done, you've overcome the first hurdle.

One thing that has emerged during the course of the experiment is that losing weight is not just about picking the right diet. Of course, many of the more sensible diets out there can help you lose weight and different ones are better for different people – that's one of the things that this book looks into, helping you find the best kind of weight-loss programme for your needs. But, however good the diet, sad to say, you won't lose weight if you don't approach dieting in the right way. You must believe that you can control your weight. The diet can help, but 'it' can't do it for you. You need to have the right mental approach, to be realistic about what you can achieve and to look at your lifestyle so that every area of your life is geared up towards losing weight. It sounds like a lot of work, but I really hope that with this book to guide you, you'll find it's a lot easier than you think.

The basis of the book is a six-step guide to the skills you need to lose weight and keep it off. Starting with whether you're mentally ready to lose weight, through setting yourself goals and learning what constitutes a healthy diet, to looking at the different diets around you and working out which ones might work for you, there's everything here to help you diet successfully. There are some eating plans too – yes, I know, the tendency is to flick straight to them, but please don't, you'll benefit from them much more if you work through the earlier chapters first, believe me.

To present *Diet Trials* I only had to observe – not to diet. In fact the producers actively discouraged me from participating (thank god) so that the attention was on all of the diets and not just one (which may or may not have worked for me). Now, though, I look forward as much as you do, to digesting the results – and hopefully little else – in the months ahead.

s e

the basics

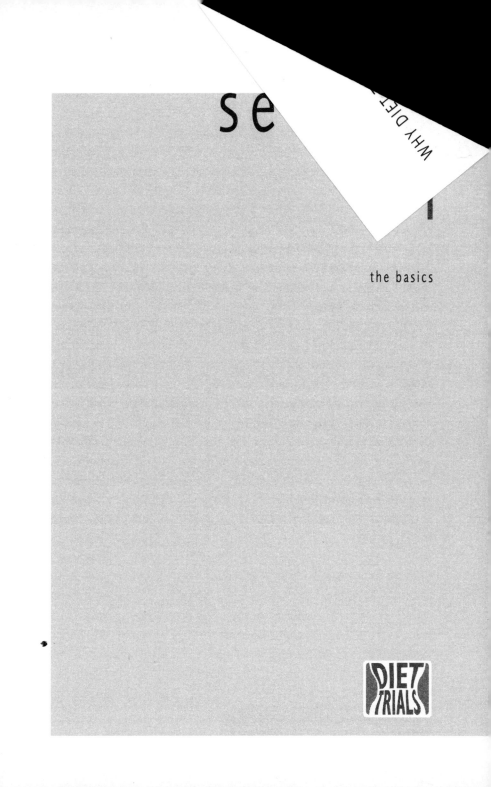

DIET
TRIALS

Obesity is set to become our biggest health problem. In the UK alone, over half of all adults are now overweight and one in five is obese (at least 13–19 kg/2–3 stone overweight). And based upon the trend, in a few years that will increase to one in four.

OK, so we're getting fatter – why should we worry? The simple reason is that it can stop us living life to the full. Carrying too much extra weight is not a cosmetic issue. Far from it. Obesity shaves an average nine years from our lifespans. Yes, I did just say nine years!

And since studies suggest that two-thirds of British adults are currently either 'watching' their weight or actively trying to lose some, you too are likely to be concerned about your weight and want to control it as best you can. Helpful advice is available from your local doctor or dietitian, but services can be limited. Then there's the vast range of commercial weight-loss approaches – books, magazines, the Internet, slimming clubs, meal replacements, health clubs, patches and potions. While some are obviously at best a laugh or at worst a demoralizing rip-off, others show much promise. But there is very little research to say how effective and helpful they really are. The BBC has been working to address this by testing out popular diets that millions of us try every year.

So why *Diet Trials* – yet another diet book? Surely, it's all been said and done before? Yes, there are books that tell us how to restrict fat, cut out carbohydrates, avoid food combinations or drink endless bowls of smelly soup. But they only scrape the surface of what's really going on. If we follow one-dimensional approaches we are doomed to fail once the heady rush of the 'new diet' is over. Then there are the mounds of misleading nutritional nonsense and endless dieting myths to wade through. Trying to stay slim in an increasingly fat world can bring its own complications too; comfort and disordered eating are the worrying consequences.

We need skills to survive in this new 'toxic' environment, and *Diet Trials* will be the first book to teach them. Skills that are based on scientific studies and the most up-to-date information we have about what best helps people lose weight, and most importantly keep it off. Skills we can pass on to our children by being positive role models. Skills to help us get out of – or avoid entering – the diet cycle and achieve the long-term success we crave, and need, for our overall health and well-being.

Diet Trials will

- ☐ Help you understand why so many people are now overweight.
- ☐ Provide information about the health consequences of being overweight or obese.
- ☐ Explain that weight problems are actually quite complex, but can be managed.
- ☐ Combat judgmental attitudes about weight.
- ☐ Help you decide if and why you need to lose weight.
- ☐ Help you to sort good advice from the bad.
- ☐ Provide you with the motivation for change, together with the skills and confidence to work out how to best manage your weight – for life.

WHY WORRY ABOUT OUR WEIGHT?

Do you worry about your weight? Has your doctor advised you to lose weight for your health's sake, but you're at a loss about how to do it? Are you alarmed by the fact that over the years your weight keeps creeping up? Are you fed up with yo-yo dieting?

If you said yes to any of these questions, you're not alone. Some people constantly worry about their weight. And most of us have tried to lose weight at some time. In fact, studies suggest that one in three will be doing so right now. Weight and body-shape are two of life's more sensitive and tricky issues. Few of us like to talk about what we weigh, and few of us are happy with how we look. Too often we strive to be an 'ideal' weight or acquire a different physique. But it's neither natural – nor healthy – for us to look like male or female supermodels. We are all different shapes and sizes, and what is natural is our own unique personality and appearance.

That said, there are real health risks linked to being overweight, especially if you are 13–19kg (2–3 stone), or more, overweight (known as 'obesity', see page 20). While we can't change our basic body shape, we *can* control how fat and fit we are. This doesn't mean that we have to be superslim, but it does make sense to aim to keep to a weight that is healthy, and feels comfortable. A weight where we have the energy and ability to fully enjoy a long life, and the pleasures it brings.

Until relatively recently, weight and shape were largely seen as things that have an impact on our appearance, and how well we fit into our clothes. But there is now a very powerful body of research that spells out just how dangerous obesity is for our health.

The fact that obesity has tripled in the last 20 years, and over half of all adults, as well as one in five children are overweight, makes the problem even more compelling. Perhaps one of the most alarming signs is that obesity-linked type 2 diabetes, a disease that once only affected adults over 40, is appearing in children and teenagers. A trend that has alarmed international obesity experts enough to announce that we may have the first generation of children to be outlived by their parents.

Obesity is now the commonest cause of ill health in the UK, and a recent report by the National Audit Office concluded that, on average, it shaves nine years off our lifespan. So health professionals' concerns and responses to the increasing weight of the nation is not because we are 'fat-fascists', but because we have seen the enormous impact obesity can have on the health and well-being of people of all ages. Sadly and unfairly obesity can affect not just health, but quality of life through limited mobility and isolation, as well as through social and job discrimination. So much of this can be prevented if people have the skills to cope with the toxic environment we now live in – and the complex medical condition that we now recognize obesity to be.

Being overweight and obese can increase the risk and/or the severity of many illnesses and problems. Some of them are:

- Insulin resistance and Syndrome X (see page 14)
- High blood pressure
- Type 2 diabetes
- Coronary heart disease
- Heart failure
- Stroke
- Raised 'bad' LDL cholesterol levels
- Raised blood triglyceride levels (a type of fat linked to heart disease)
- Certain cancers, especially colon, prostate, ovarian and postmenopausal breast cancer
- Gall bladder disease
- Back pain
- Infertility, irregular periods
- Polycystic ovarian syndrome (PCOS)
- Pregnancy complications such as gestational diabetes, high blood pressure and early labour
- Depression
- Low self-esteem and social isolation
- Osteoarthritis, joint pain
- Lower resistance to infections, including the common cold
- Stress incontinence
- Breathlessness
- Asthma
- Excessive sweating
- Sleep difficulties, including sleep apnoea (see page 25)
- Incontinence
- Complications during surgery, anaesthetic risk

THE TOXIC ENVIRONMENT

We gain weight if we take in more calories than we burn. It's that simple. Many of us will gain around a pound a year without realizing it. Some of us will gain a lot more. It's not because we are greedy, bad or even obviously overeating. It's because we live in an environment where food is everywhere and activity is discouraged. A place where food is so abundant that eating purely for hunger is a rarity rather than a given.

Not only is food convenient (think fast-food chains, chocolates and crisps at tills), it's seductively advertised, quickly prepared, cheap, confusingly labelled, in big-portion sizes and tastes better than ever. Meanwhile, we sit at desks, in front of television and computer screens or behind a steering wheel.

In evolutionary terms our bodies are not ready for this constant feast and sloth. We used to search, hunt and dig for food; now we drive to supermarkets, heat and serve. And because food is so accessible, it's something we can readily use to cope with life's stresses. So we snack, graze and eat more than our bodies need to keep to a healthy weight, without even realizing it.

There have been lots of other theories to try and explain the

Insulin Resistance and Syndrome X

Insulin resistance is thought to affect around one in five adults in the UK, but most aren't aware of it. It is a condition where the body cells stop responding properly to the action of the hormone insulin. This prompts the pancreas (which produces insulin) to pump more of the hormone into the bloodstream – but the insulin still struggles to work effectively – and eventually the cells ignore it altogether. Having too much insulin circulating in the blood is bad news. It can raise levels of blood sugar (glucose), cholesterol and triglycerides – another type of fat – in the blood. It can cause high blood pressure and release too much of the stress hormone cortisol –

which can depress immunity. Over time, it can lead to type 2 diabetes, probably because the insulin-producing beta cells in the pancreas simply wear out.

There seems to be a genetic tendency for insulin resistance. But carrying too much excess body fat, especially around your middle (apple shaped or a beer belly) is the biggest risk factor. The bottom line is that having too much fat around your waist (see page 22) can prevent insulin from working properly.

Insulin resistance is the underlying cause of Syndrome X. This means that people with the condition tend to be apple shaped and suffer from the sorts of health problems listed on page 13.

fattening of the nation. Food intolerance, pesticides, infections, sugar and genetic changes are just some. But the research keeps telling us again and again that we now find it hard not to consume more calories than we burn, thanks to the environment we live in. Our genes, for example, can't solely be to blame, because obesity has increased massively in the past 20 years – and there is no way our gene pool could change in that time!

What we do have is food to buy on every street corner. Food manufacturers advertise indulgence. Celebrity chefs entice us to pour in the cream and olive oil. Supermarkets offer more and more quickly prepared meals and treats. Food and drink is the centre of social events. We eat out more than ever or dial for a delivery. We enjoy a drink, which stimulates appetite and 'dissolves' good intentions. We are lured by the promise of 'low-fat' foods without realizing that added sugars mean they aren't also low-calorie. We eat more than we want thanks to tempting 'meal deals' and 'all you can eat' offers.

But surely we 'need' this convenience? After all, we are busy people with less time to cook. In reality, we rush so much we have no time for exercise. When we're not rushing we make use of labour- and energy-saving remote controls, lifts and escalators, washing machines, automatic car-washes, central heating. In fact, it is estimated that our energy output has declined by 30 per cent since the rise of the toxic environment. Studies in the USA suggest that watching television may be one of the most important factors behind childhood and adolescent obesity. This is hardly surprising when, on average, children watch 28 hours a week – which means they would burn nearly 600 calories a day less than children who spent that time playing outside instead. Watching TV doesn't just mean that children are inactive rather than involved in active play. It can also promote high-fat snacking – especially with all the advertisements fired at them.

And then there's our genetic inheritance from our hunter-gatherer ancestors. All those tens of thousands of years ago food was often in scarce supply so they ate as much as they could when they had it, to store fat ready for leaner times. This means we still have a strong hunger drive even if we are overweight – our genes still think we can't afford to take the risk of missing out! Annoyingly, these 'drive to eat' mechanisms aren't as efficient when it comes to stopping eating – so we can happily go-ahead and eat whether we are hungry or not.

The Story of the Pima Indians

One real-life example of how the toxic environment has taken a grip on the lives and health of modern man, who evolved from hunter-gatherers, is the story of the American Pima Indians. There are two groups of Pima Indians who share the same gene pool. Today, one group lives on an accessible reservation in Arizona, the other in the very isolated Sierra Madre mountains of Mexico. When nutritionists studied the health of both groups, they found that the Arizona Indians, who had easy access to a refined US diet and no reason to be active, were very overweight and suffered much ill health; over half had diabetes and gall bladder disease for example. Meanwhile, the mountain-dwelling Indians, who follow a traditional, unrefined, low-fat diet had very few 'western' diseases, including obesity and diabetes.

To counteract the toxic environment we don't need to face limited food supplies or become athletes. Small and subtle changes to our lifestyle can be enough to tip the balance in our favour so that our weight stays more or less stable over the years, rather than gradually (or sometimes rapidly) climbing. And active living plus a healthy diet don't just help to control our weight, but can also boost our health in all sorts of ways. Regular exercise helps combat stress and low moods; good nutrition boosts our overall well-being and cuts our risk of long-term problems such as heart disease, cancers, bowel disorders and osteoporosis.

Big Food Means Big Waistlines?

Have you noticed how portion sizes have got bigger? According to recent research from the USA, this could be one of the chief reasons why so many people find it so hard to manage their weight. The study compared food portion sizes in the 1970s from fast-food outlets and family-type restaurants, to today's portion sizes. These are the sort of places that are now coming under fire from the public (who blame them for making them obese) and that are serving the sort of high-fat food that officials are actually now considering taxing in a bid to control excessive consumption of them in the USA.

The study found that in 30 years the number of large-size portions had increased tenfold. Most foods were sold in larger amounts than recommended by government health standards. For example, pasta servings were almost five times bigger, the average muffin was the same as three 1970s' muffins, chocolate chip cookies were seven times as large and steak over twice the size!

Things aren't much better in the UK. A standard bag of crisps used to be 25g – now it's closer to 35g or sometimes 40g. If you usually ate a packet of crisps every day, the bigger portion size means you would unwittingly gain 2.5kg (5lb) in a year. 'Going large' on a cheeseburger

Calories no longer used after 50 years of labour-saving devices.

	1950s/2000s
Per week	
Shopping on foot/car and supermarket trolley	2400/276
Washing clothes by hand/machine	1500/270
Making a coal fire/lighting a gas fire	1300/Almost zero
Making a bed with blankets/duvet	575/300
Per hour	
Mowing lawn by hand mower/electric mower	500/180
Driving without power steering/with it per hour	96/75

with fries and cola will add another 165 calories and 5g fat.

Big portions are on offer because they're relatively cheap for the food industry to achieve, and it makes us feel that we're getting good value for money. So we end up being seduced by quantity rather than quality. Studies also show that food eaten away from home is higher in fat. And we eat more than we normally do when we're served large portions – and quickly get used to those big-portion sizes. Then, when we cook at home, we want more food to keep us satisfied.

Quick-Fix Diets and Potions

Since so many of us are overweight, and are trying to do something about it, there's a vast diet industry out there trying to sell us that help. As you will see in Section Three, some sectors are much more helpful, and honest, than others. Metabolism myths and downright nonsense abound, making it confusing for people to have confidence in their ability to control their weight.

This misinformation is all part of the toxic environment. The less scrupulous elements of the diet industry offer short-term 'solutions' to a long-term issue, without giving a thought to the impact their wares may have on our physical and mental well-being. But when people feel desperate the lure of easy and permanent weight loss is too tempting to overlook. Then there are crash diets that drastically restrict what and how much you eat. Sure, they will help you lose weight quickly (although much of this is fluid), but they can't be sustained. The diet is soon broken, the weight is regained and you, the innocent victim, feel a failure. When, in fact, the cranky diet failed you.

All of this dieting 'noise' detracts us from the real issues. Achieving and maintaining a healthy weight relies on sustainable lifestyle changes that suit your individual needs. They must be changes that you want to make, and changes that you can continue with. This all takes some time, reflection and commitment. In short, the quick-fix won't work.

WHAT IS A HEALTHY WEIGHT?

The logical answer to the question 'What is a healthy weight?' is any weight at which you feel good, have the energy to do what you want to do, enjoy a varied diet and have no weight-related medical problems. In other words, the weight at which you are healthy and comfortable. We now know that there is no single ideal weight for any one person. We also know that it's not just about carrying too much fat – where that fat is stored has a big influence on our health. As does our body composition. Some people may weigh more than others because they are active enough to develop larger muscles, and their body fat is in fact at a healthy level.

Body Fat

While having too much extra body fat is not good for us, we still need a fair amount to stay well and healthy. Body fat (known as 'adipose tissue') isn't just inert lumps of fat. It has its own blood supply and releases and regulates hormones in the body. For example, body fat is needed to produce optimal levels of the female hormone, oestrogen. If the proportion of fat in a woman's body drops too low (below 18 per cent) oestrogen levels plummet, sex drive wanes, periods stop, fertility declines, bones weaken and blood cholesterol rises. This is the main reason why women of childbearing age tend to be pear shaped (see page 22). All those hip and thigh fat deposits are there to keep us in tip-top reproductive shape. Body fat also provides a cushion for bones and kidneys, and acts as an energy reserve in case we fall very ill or, heaven forbid, go short of food.

The Body Mass Index Explained

The Body Mass Index (BMI) is currently the internationally accepted standard for assessing how healthy, or otherwise, our weight is.

You have no doubt seen BMI height–weight charts in magazines or your doctor's surgery, and had a look to see which range or coloured band you fit in to. If you prefer maths, you may have even worked out your BMI – your weight (in kilograms) divided by your height (in metres) squared.

For example, the BMI of a 72kg (11 stone 5lb) woman who is 1.64m (5ft 5in) tall is: 72 divided by (1.64 x 1.64) = 26.8.

The World Health Organization and UK health experts use the following BMI ranges:

- Underweight: less than 18.5
- Healthy weight: 18.5–24.9
- Overweight: 25–29.9
- Obese: 30–34.9
- Very obese: 35–39.9
- Extremely obese: 40 or more

Note: Please seek medical advice if your BMI is greater than 35, as you are likely to have medical problems and may need additional help with managing your weight and health.

Health and the BMI

Adults within the 'healthy weight' range have the lowest risk of ill health. 'Overweight' carries only a little increased risk, but this increases markedly if you also smoke or have other health problems (see below). Once people fall into the BMI ranges of 30 to 40 or more they are at a very high risk of health problems such as type 2 diabetes, coronary heart disease; certain cancers and osteoarthritis (also see page 13).

People in the 'underweight' range are also at increased risk of health problems, for example, infertility, osteoporosis (brittle bones), lower resistance to infection and slower recovery from illness. It may also be a sign that they have an eating disorder. But some people are naturally slender, and are quite healthy in the upper levels of this range.

The BMI, however, is not so accurate for very muscled people as it can push them into a higher BMI category, despite having a healthy level of body fat (true underweight can also be masked, as muscle can make people appear 'healthy' when they actually have unhealthily low levels of body fat).

Also, within any BMI range, risk to health for an individual can vary according to a number of factors including age, sex, whether they smoke, level of physical activity, fat distribution and other illnesses such as diabetes, joint problems or high blood pressure. For example, smoking increases health risks at all BMI ranges, while overweight people who are physically fit and active may have a reduced risk of dying from coronary heart disease compared to unfit, inactive people in the healthy weight range.

Waist Measurements

Another recognized way to assess your weight is to check your fat distribution with a waist measurement. It's important to do this because more fat around your abdomen – often referred to as being apple shaped or having the classic 'beer belly' – carries significantly greater health risks than excess fat around the hips (known as being pear shaped).

A high waist measurement also means you're more likely to have too much fat lying around in your blood. This is bad news because it increases your risk of insulin resistance, high blood pressure, raised cholesterol and type 2 diabetes. Even if you are slim in other places, if your waist measurement is too high (see below) then some 'waist loss' makes sense for your health's sake. It can also help you feel fitter and more agile – in more ways than one...

Men are more commonly apple shaped and women tend to be pear shaped, but after the hormonal changes of the menopause, fat distribution changes and women become more apple shaped. This also means we take on apple shaped health risks. Cigarette smoking, drinking too much alcohol and lack of physical activity are also linked to laying down more fat around your middle. One thing to note, though, is that your basic body shape is inherited and can't really be changed. So if you come from a long line of 'pears', losing weight will mean you become a smaller, trimmer and healthier pear.

Measuring your waist is quite straightforward. Use a tape measure (it might be easier if you get someone to help you) and measure your waist at the belly-button level. Men should make sure they don't measure around where their belt goes, as it tends to work its way down and sit below bulbous bellies. This can make it seem as though your waist size hasn't increased, despite the loss of your six pack! For women 32–34¾in (81–88cm) indicates 'increasing health risk' and further weight/waist increases should be avoided (or some lost). 35 inches (88cm) or more indicates 'high risk' and weight/waist loss is advised For men 37–39¾in (94–102cm) indicates 'increasing health risk' and 40in (102cm) or more indicates 'high risk'.

Measuring Body Fat

Measuring body fat is especially useful when regular exercise is a key part of your approach to weight control. As well as seeing how the scales change, you can assess how the amount of fat in your body changes. And since muscle weighs more than fat, this can encouragingly show that you may be doing better than you think! Body fat can be measured in a number of ways.

DXA Scans

All the subjects in *Diet Trials* had DXA (dual energy X-ray absorptiometry) scans carried out at the start and the end of the six-month study period. This is one of the best ways to assess changes in body composition – that is, how the amount of fat and lean tissue (muscle) in their bodies changed over six months. It was originally developed to measure bone and is widely used to diagnose osteoporosis. It is also able to give a guide to how fat is distributed throughout the body, for example, in the arms and legs relative to the abdomen.

It was important in helping to assess whether some of the diet programmes were better at conserving muscle and bone strength and promoting fat loss than others – and in checking that some of the weight loss wasn't due to lots of fluid loss, rather than fat loss.

Skin-fold Measurements

Skinfold thicknesses are often measured at health clubs, usually at four specific sites on the body. From these measurements the amount of fat in the whole body can be estimated. It's important to ensure that the person doing the test is experienced as this helps the measurement to be more accurate – although it, and the method below, can never be as accurate as DXA.

Bioelectrical Impedance

Bioelectrical Impedance (BIA) is another simple way of assessing body composition and it may be used at health clubs or by your doctor. It involves attaching four electrodes to the hand and foot on one side of the body. Simpler still, and something that can be used at home, are bathroom scales with inbuilt BIA facilities. Hand-held versions are also available.

While the BIA and skinfold methods aren't as accurate as more complex ones such as the DXA scan, they will at least give you more of an idea of the amount of fat in your body, than commonly used weighing scales or the BMI alone can give you.

WHAT ARE THE BENEFITS OF LOSING WEIGHT?

By now you've probably got the picture that being overweight or obese can affect your health. But all of us like to do things for a reason; so, does losing weight make us healthier?

The simple answer is 'yes'. The even better news is that you don't have to get down to an 'ideal' or 'model slim' weight to reap the benefits. Research is now clear that modest weight loss, that is losing just 5 to 10 per cent of your body weight, leads to big health benefits. Here's a motivating example.

For someone who weighs 100kg (about 15½ stone), losing 10kg (1½ stone), which is 10 per cent of their body weight, could result in at least a:

- 20 per cent reduction in the risk of dying from any cause
- 30 per cent reduction in the risk of dying from diabetes-related problems
- 40 per cent reduction in the risk of dying from an obesity-related cancer
- 10 mmHG drop in systolic blood pressure (the first, and higher number)

- 20 mmHG drop in diastolic blood pressure (the second number)
- 50 per cent fall in blood glucose levels – measured when fasting
- 10 per cent drop in blood cholesterol
- 30 per cent drop in blood triglycerides (raised levels may be as big a risk factor for heart disease as raised cholesterol levels)

This sort of modest weight loss also greatly improves insulin resistance, and alleviates problems such as joint pain, breathlessness, low moods and sleep apnoea (when people stop breathing for very short periods during sleep). It has also been shown to improve menstruation and fertility problems, including those linked with polycystic ovarian syndrome (PCOS).

Encouragingly, modest weight loss amongst women can reduce depressive symptoms and binge eating rather than make things worse – a common concern when people try to restrict what they eat (read more about the psychological effects of dieting in Section Two).

Weight Control During Pregnancy

There are times in our lives when weight loss is not recommended, and during pregnancy is definitely one of them. However, a healthy level of weight gain is sensible as excessive gains can increase the risk of high blood pressure, gestational diabetes and health problems for the baby. Nor is it wise to be dieting if you're trying to have a baby. You need to be as well nourished as possible when you conceive, as well as during pregnancy. If you are very overweight, it makes sense to get to a healthier weight before trying for a baby.

What if Your Weight Just Stays the Same?

Thanks to our toxic environment, most of us are gradually gaining weight. So just managing to keep your weight stable is a notable achievement. It shows that you have developed skills that enable you to survive and not get ensnared by the environment's food, inactivity, comfort eating and quick-fix diet traps.

Research strongly suggests that people who stay a stable weight, even if they are moderately overweight, stay healthier than those whose weight fluctuates. Studies have also compared 'health centred' non-diet approaches to helping people to eat healthily, be active, get in touch with natural hunger and fullness and enhance body acceptance with more traditional 'weight-loss centred' programmes. While the latter lead to better weight loss, both approaches improve physical and emotional well-being. This reinforces the general health benefits of a healthy lifestyle and attitude.

Long-term weight control needs the skills and confidence to make lifestyle changes, which include setting realistic weight goals. *Diet Trials* will help you develop these skills as well as help you to sort the good diets from the bad.

WHAT MAKES US GAIN WEIGHT?

'More in than out and you're stout!'

While the reasons for weight gain are simple, there is nothing simple about controlling our weight – especially now that we live in such a toxic environment. We all have different lifestyles, appetites, family experiences, food preferences, activity levels, budgets, stresses,

Modest weight loss halves risk of type 2 diabetes

Type 2 diabetes develops when the amount of glucose (sugar) in the blood is persistently too high because the body can't use it properly. Symptoms include excessive thirst, blurred vision, frequent trips to the loo and tiredness. It's known to affect more than two per cent of the UK population, but the true incidence may be much higher. It usually develops in middle age (but is now appearing in children) and being very overweight is a major cause. Proper treatment helps to reduce the high risk of heart disease and eye, kidney and nerve problems that are commonly caused by diabetes.

Recent research in the USA and Finland has found that people at high risk of developing diabetes can more than halve this risk through small but effective changes to diet such as eating less fat and more fruit and vegetables, combined with 30 minutes of daily exercise, such as walking. These changes also helped participants to lose modest amounts of weight – about 3kg to 4kg (half a stone) on average – and this was enough to make a life-enhancing difference.

relationships with food and health problems. But despite these unique complexities (and despite what 'fad' diet approaches might tell you), weight-control regulation ultimately comes down to one simple equation. The equation of energy balance: energy intake (from food and drink) versus energy output (calories burned via metabolism and activity). When these two are in balance, our weight remains stable. 'Calories' is the term used to describe the energy content of food. When we consume more calories than we burn we gain weight; and when we consume less than we burn, we lose it.

Fortunately, the body is a wonderfully designed structure; constantly conducting automatic, regulatory checks and balances on its life-sustaining processes. So, in the right environment, we would be pretty good at matching calorie intake and output, and staying at a healthy weight. But put us in today's toxic environment – where our natural regulatory systems are easily overridden – and things start to go awry. Life events such as having a baby, a new job, retiring, emotional upsets or illness also have a major impact. And even small changes can make a difference. Consistently eating a mere 50 calories (one plain biscuit) extra a day could lead to a 2.3kg (5lb) weight gain in a year.

When you think about it, it's amazing that anyone does stay slim these days – finding out how slim people survive the toxic environment is certainly something worth doing! But the fact that small changes in the wrong direction spells weight gain means we only need to make small changes in the right direction to tip the balance in our favour.

What Makes Us Eat?

Surely we eat because we're hungry? Or maybe it's because we like the look of something? Then again, it could be because we're stressed and food brings some relief? When we think about it we actually eat for all sorts of reasons. Not to mention for the pure pleasure of it.

The hypothalamus in the brain appears to be the chief control centre of our drive to eat. It takes account of messages from nerves and hormones, coming from other parts of the brain as well as from the mouth, stomach, intestines, fat cells and liver, as to how much we've recently eaten, how much energy we've burnt and how much we've stored. Physical, stomach-rumbling and gnawing hunger provides our most basic drive to eat. Our general interest and appetite for, the food in front of us is also involved. Feelings of fullness tell us when to stop eating, and feelings of satisfaction keep us from wanting to eat between meals.

Of course, if eating was that well controlled none of us would have a weight problem. Internal or external triggers, such as emotions or a sumptuous buffet (see page 139), can override these 'internal regulators'. Eating can also be suppressed by emotion, or by consciously defying our innate drive to eat – as in strict dieting or in eating disorders.

Food As Fuel

Food is made up of carbohydrates, fats, proteins, fibre, vitamins, minerals and water. Energy in food, which is measured in calories or kilojoules, is mainly supplied by carbohydrates (sugars and starches), fats, proteins and alcohol. Fat contains more than twice the calories of protein or carbohydrate (and makes food taste good), which is why it's so 'fattening'. Vitamins and minerals help the body release energy from food. It uses this energy for every metabolic function – breathing, digesting food, brain, nerve and muscle function, heartbeats, temperature regulation, immunity – as well as physical activity.

If we take in more calories from fat than we need to fuel our day-to-day energy needs, we store the excess in fat cells or 'adipose tissue'. If we overfeed the cells enough, these fat stores can just keep on growing (both their size and number can increase).

When it comes to carbohydrates, we can store a limited amount in the liver and muscles. These carbohydrate stores are known as 'glycogen'. They are used to keep blood glucose levels topped up between meals and act as a direct source of fuel for moving muscles. The vast majority

Energy Output

There are three main parts to the energy we expend or burn:

- Resting metabolic rate (RMR): the amount of energy we expend when we are lying down and resting. This usually accounts for around two-thirds of all the calories we burn each day. Our weight has the biggest influence on how high our RMR will be – the heavier we are, the higher it is. We can also calculate our RMR with equations (see page 104). The only way to increase RMR – and then only mildly – is to increase how much muscle we have (relative to fat), with regular exercise.
- Thermogenesis: the energy used to keep warm, digest food and respond to stress. This is typically around 10 per cent of calories burnt, and is fairly constant.
- Physical activity: this includes all movement, not just sport or conscious exercise. It burns the remaining calories and is the most flexible part of our energy output. The more active we are the more calories we burn – and physically active people tend to have lower body-fat levels than inactive people.

of the remaining carbohydrate is used directly for energy – and not stored as body fat – as is often claimed by some popular diet books. Rats can do this, but we humans aren't very good at it.

We can't store any alcohol at all, since it serves no useful purpose in the body. This means it's immediately used as fuel allowing the other nutrients in a meal, fat in particular, to be stored – usually in the 'ready and waiting' fat cells in the abdomen. Maybe this helps to explain beer bellies!

While protein can be a source of fuel, the body prefers to harness it to build new body proteins, which are used for growth, repair of normal wear and tear, and regulation of bodily processes. If we eat a lot of protein and not much carbohydrate – as we might if we follow a high protein, low carbohydrate diet – then it can be used for energy, along with protein in muscle and other body tissues (known as 'lean tissue'). This lean tissue can be broken down to produce glucose to maintain vital blood glucose (sugar) levels and so compensate for low levels of carbohydrate in the diet.

High-Risk Times and Situations for Weight Gain

- **Childhood** Childhood is a time when eating patterns and food preferences are formed. While not all overweight children become obese adults their risk is increased, especially if a child stays, or becomes, overweight as he or she gets older. And the more overweight a child is, the more likely they are to remain overweight or obese as they become adults. Young children are at most risk of becoming obese adults if they have obese parents. In fact, children with two obese parents have about a 70 per cent risk of becoming obese compared to less than 20 per cent for children with two parents who are healthy weights.
- **Leaving home** Gone are home-cooked meals, or at least a regular and free supply of healthy food in the fridge. Busy lifestyles, a lack of cooking skills and tight budgets often mean convenience food grabbed on the run or a visit to the chippy on the way home from the pub! This

style of eating means diets are likely to be high in fat and low in fruits and vegetables; a combination which makes it easy to overeat without realising it – until the pounds start to creep on....

- **Marriage/moving in together** Food and love go together, whether it's romantic meals out, home-cooked treats, or shared wine and chocolate over a good video. Living together may also result in stopping healthy habits like playing sport or going to the gym. Initially, couples are usually more interested in pleasing and indulging each other than in worrying about keeping up a healthy lifestyle! A lack of knowledge about choosing a healthy diet and how to cook also has an impact. And don't forget that women typically need fewer calories than men, so take care not to serve the same amount for both of you.

- **Stopping smoking** If you smoke, the best thing you can do for your health is give up. It's far more dangerous to smoke than be overweight; in fact, you would need to gain 20kg (3 stone 2lb) before the health gain of not smoking is cancelled out. Not only is smoking strongly linked to heart disease and cancer, it also increases the risk of osteoporosis (brittle bones) and problems during pregnancy. Worryingly, four in 10 women use smoking as a weight control method.

- **Pregnancy** Gaining a certain level of extra weight is all part of a healthy pregnancy, but failing to lose it afterwards is the most common reason

Calories in food

Calories come from the following nutrients. Note how high the calorie count is in fat and alcohol compared to protein and carbohydrate. Eating less fat is therefore a useful way to cut calories.

Carbohydrate : 4 calories per gram

Protein: 4 calories per gram

Fat: 9 calories per gram

Alcohol: 7 calories per gram

obese women give as the cause of their problem. On average, pregnant women lay down about 4kg (9lb) of extra fat. This is nature's way of providing a reserve to meet the additional calorie needs of pregnancy and breastfeeding. Studies show that there is no physical reason why losing weight after having a baby should be more difficult than losing it at any other time. It seems to be mainly due to the big changes in diet and lifestyle that go hand in hand with having a baby. But it is possible to get back to a healthier weight by eating wisely and being as active as you can. It just takes around 12 months on average, which is longer than many women think – or would like!

■ **Menopause** While research shows that there is no real slump in metabolism after the menopause, women often state that this a time when they gain weight, especially if they start hormone replacement therapy (HRT). However, a three-year study found that menopausal women taking HRT gained less weight than those who didn't. Again, lifestyle changes appear to be the most likely cause of weight gain. But remember that the hormonal changes of the menopause do cause a change in where fat is distributed in the body (see page 22).

■ **Retirement** Many people gain weight after retirement due to a change in the pace of their lifestyle: less stress, more time to relax, watch television, cook and eat. On the other hand, some find they use their extra time to get fitter and slimmer. What a good idea!

■ **Getting older** The statistics show that as a nation we get fatter as we get older. For example, around 10 per cent of 16 to 24 year olds are obese compared to 30 per cent of people aged 55 to 64 years. But it doesn't have to be like that. Yes, there is a small decrease in our metabolic rate as we age (about 5 per cent per decade), but the main reason for weight gain is that people generally become less active and lose metabolism-maintaining muscle strength. Only a small number regularly take part in active pursuits like swimming, gardening, dancing, golf or bowls. At the same time, there isn't a similar decline in the amount they eat – so the excess energy is stored as fat!

■ **Emotional responses to food** Using food to cope with stress and emotional ups and downs is a common reason for overeating, not to mention gaining weight or thwarting weight-loss progress. If you feel that emotional eating is one of your problems there are ways to overcome it and get back in control (see page 141).

HOW DO WE LOSE WEIGHT – AND KEEP IT OFF?

You've heard all about how the nation is getting fatter, that obesity is bad for your health, that a toxic environment is largely to blame, that you need skills to survive it – and that fad and quick-fix diets won't help. So I guess you're wondering how on earth you do control your weight? Read *Diet Trials* and you will learn the required survival skills. You will also discover more about the real science behind weight, health and weight loss.

Weight Loss – the Facts

Despite claims to the contrary by popular diet books and self-styled gurus, calories do count and we only lose weight when we consume fewer calories than we burn.

Our weight typically fluctuates by a few pounds on a day-to-day basis. You'll know that scary feeling when you weigh yourself in the morning then again at night, or after a meal out, and it looks like you've gained pounds in a day. But this is largely due to fluid changes and is not a reflection of body fat fluctuations. Don't be fooled either by what seems to very rapid weight loss in the first week or so of quick-fix or low-carbohydrate diets. This is mainly caused by fluid loss. When we first cut our calorie and carbohydrate intake right back, we use up the body's carbohydrate (glycogen) stores in the liver and muscles. Glycogen is stored with three times its weight in water, meaning that 2kg to 3kg (4½lb to just over 6½lb) losses are possible. However, these losses are just as rapidly reversed when we eat a large meal or return to our usual eating habits and refill our glycogen stores.

True weight change happens over longer periods of time, which is why losing weight – or indeed gaining it – is a long-term process that involves sustained and conscious changes to our usual eating habits and the amount of exercise we take.

Calories Do Count

Food and drink provide the calories and nutrients we need to stay well, healthy and energetic. Our individual calorie needs vary according to our weight, age, sex and activity level, but on average, women require around 2000 calories a day to stay in energy balance and so keep their weight stable. Men need around 2500 a day. Overweight and/or very active people will need more to stay in energy balance.

The energy content of 0.5kg (1lb 1oz) of stored body fat is 3500 calories. So to lose 0.5kg (1lb 1oz) a week, a 500 calorie 'deficit' is needed each day ($7 \times 500 = 3500$). We can achieve this by consuming fewer calories, by being extremely active – or, ideally, by doing a bit of both.

So, if someone normally burns around 2300 calories a day, they will lose about a pound a week if they reduce their daily intake to 1800 calories. If they also build in a 30-minute brisk walk (which burns 120–150 calories) each day, they will lose just over a pound a week.

Healthy Weight Loss

When we lose weight, it's important that we do it in a healthy way to ensure that we continue to enjoy food, get all the nutrients we need, can get on with our lives, feel positive about helping our health and improve our body composition (lose fat and optimize muscle).

This approach means that we don't just follow a weight-loss diet, but develop new skills and attitudes to help us keep the weight off. It's obvious, then, that short-term and one-dimensional diet plans or workouts aren't going to be enough. What the research – and successful slimmers – tell us is that a combination of approaches is vital: a healthy diet, being more active and a change in day-to-day thoughts and behaviours.

And all three have to be kept up, literally, for life. Hopefully, government, schools, workplaces and the food industry will work together to make the healthy choice the easier choice. But some people with more complex problems may also benefit from anti-obesity drugs, or surgery if they are severely obese and have tried all the conventional approaches.

Most importantly, you have to find what works best for you. You will hopefully glean new and helpful information from this book, and combine it with other experiences and knowledge that also help. The best plan of action is not simply to aim to get to a certain weight, but to work at identifying why you have difficulties getting to or maintaining a healthy weight. Couple this with the belief that you can manage your weight, and with the aspiration to develop personal skills to achieve your goals, and there'll be no going back. There is no single 'right' way for you, or anyone else, to control your weight. You have to solve that jigsaw for yourself. *Diet Trials* will help you to find the pieces that suit your needs, and will help you put them together.

Exploding Myths About Weight Loss and Diets

'Knowledge is power', the old saying goes. While science certainly doesn't have all the answers, we certainly know enough to stamp out ongoing myths that only serve to undermine confidence in your abilities.

1   Food eaten late at night is more fattening
This has been investigated and disproved by a study at an esteemed nutrition research centre in Cambridge. The results revealed that,

when total calorie intake was the same a large meal eaten late at night did not make the body store more fat than small meals eaten over the day. It's the total amount you eat in a 24-hour period that's important. But it is true that people who skip meals during the day and then eat loads in the evening are more likely to be overweight than people who balance their intake with regular meals.

2 'Low-fat' and 'fat-free' foods are low calorie

Be warned. 'Low-fat' or 'fat-free' does not necessarily mean low-calorie or calorie-free. Always check the calorie content of foods that make such claims, especially cakes, biscuits, crisps, ice creams and ready meals. Extra sugars and thickeners are often added to boost flavour and texture, so calorie content may be only a bit less than, or similar to, that of standard products. And an '85% fat free' claim means the food is actually 15 per cent fat (French fries are 85 per cent fat free!).

3 Overweight people have slow metabolisms

For a long time, a slow metabolic rate (the rate at which we burn calories) seemed like an understandable explanation for obesity. But after years of research it is now clear that people who are overweight actually have a higher metabolic rate than lighter people. This is because heavier bodies use more energy (calories) to function and move around. Differences in appetite control and spontaneous activity level, rather than metabolic rate, are now seen as being two of the main genetic factors behind obesity. But the good news is that we can control these genetic influences with a healthy diet and active lifestyle.

4 I only eat 1200 calories a day and still can't lose weight

Virtually any adult who consistently consumes this number of calories will lose weight – although different people will lose it at different rates (heavier and more active people will do so more quickly). Sometimes it may seem that you can't lose weight – and that will be because you are consuming more calories than you realize.

Research shows that it's extremely difficult to estimate how much we eat. This could be unwittingly eating bigger portion sizes than recommended, foods being higher in calories than we think, forgotten nibbles, and other forms of 'unconscious' eating. In fact, studies show that some people under-report by 800 calories a day, and forgetting 400 calories is not unusual. Interestingly, studies also show that the heavier we are, the harder we find it to be accurate about how much we eat.

5   **If you diet your metabolism drops making it hard to lose weight**
When we eat less our metabolism does decline because our body tries to conserve energy in case its food supply is about to run out. But it's not as extreme as people often think. On a 1200-calorie diet, for example, the metabolic rate only decreases by about 5 per cent. This increases to a 15 per cent drop on very low-calorie diets of less than 700 calories per day (these aren't recommended without medical advice). But despite this, there are still significant 'calorie gaps' (between calorie intake and calorie output) to promote steady weight loss. Once a significant amount of weight is lost your metabolic rate will decrease a bit because there is less of you to burn energy. You can help offset this decline by keeping up regular exercise, which helps to preserve metabolically active muscle.

6   **You can spot reduce problem areas**
Body-fat stores gain or lose fat in proportion to their size, so it's not possible to 'spot reduce' 'problem' areas. However, fat around your abdomen or waist appears to be more responsive to weight loss from diet or exercise than fat stored closer to the skin – the hips and thighs, for example. This means that with weight loss apple-shaped people with lots of fat around their waist can decrease their shape more markedly than people who are more 'pear shaped' – who will lose weight to become smaller pears. Regular exercise can tone areas of the body making them seem trimmer.

7   **Some people can eat what they like and still won't gain weight**
A large body of scientific evidence argues against this (and including the idea that these lucky people have high metabolic rates). In fact, slender people have lower resting metabolic rates than obese people because

their vital organs, including the heart, muscles, liver and digestive, tract are smaller and so need fewer calories to function. And a very carefully controlled study, which involved overfeeding slim and overweight young men by 50 per cent more than their individual calorie needs, revealed that all the subjects gained weight at the same rate.

One explanation could be that some people are more spontaneously active than others. For example, after researchers at the Mayo Clinic in the USA calculated the individual daily calorie needs of the participants in a study all the subjects were fed an additional 1000 calories each day for eight weeks. Exercise was carefully monitored and the fate of the extra 1000 calories was measured. All the participants gained weight, but the amount ranged from 2lb to almost 16lb. The researchers found that those who gained the least weight had the greatest increase in what they termed 'non-exercise activity thermogenesis' (NEAT) – this actually means twitching, fidgeting, moving around, changing posture, etc. It appeared that when some of the subjects overate, NEAT switched on and they burnt more of the excess calories.

8   Dieting makes you fat

Diets get a lot of bad press. Just the word screams 'deprivation'. Any eating plan that makes you consume fewer calories than you burn each day will lead to some weight loss. But there are a lot of bad diets out there, that are short-term and hard to 'stick to'. And while some weight might come off for a while, it usually goes back on – with a little extra – and you feel a failure. The problem is that most diets simply focus on how to eat less to lose weight, rather than how to make lifestyle changes and maintain a healthy weight. In other words, bad diets don't help to you develop the skills and confidence to lose weight and keep it off long term.

'Dieting' evolved because more and more people were becoming obese – not vice versa. It was hoped that it would be a way to cope with the effects of the toxic environment. We now know more about what survival skills are really needed.

9   All my family are obese so it's in my genes

We are all individual and have different genetic blueprints and inherited family traits – which include body shape and height. As research progresses it becomes clearer that, when people are exposed to the same toxic environment, genetic differences can make some of them more likely to stay slender, or gain weight, than others. Genetic factors relating to metabolism, control of appetite, preference for high-fat foods and levels of spontaneous physical activity may play a part in the development of weight gain. But it's not just our genes that play a role. Families usually share the same diet, lifestyle and cultural influences, and these habits tend to persist into later life.

10 I have a medical problem or genetic problem that makes it impossible to lose weight

It is actually quite rare for medical conditions or genetic problems to directly cause obesity. Thyroid disease resulting in an underactive thyroid (hypothyroidism) – which slows the metabolic rate – is the best known but, despite popular opinion, it is not an important cause of obesity. Symptoms include some weight gain, feeling the cold, a dry skin, constipation and poor concentration. Your doctor can check for hypothyroidism with a blood test, and, if the test is positive, treat the condition with medication. Women with polycystic ovarian syndrome (PCOS) suffer from insulin resistance (see page 14), and often find it more difficult to manage their weight, but it is not clear why this is.

There are some very rare genetic disorders that upset the appetite and fat storage, for example, Cushing's syndrome, Bardet Biedl syndrome, Prader-Willi syndrome and leptin deficiency (leptin is a protein that sends messages about the state of the body's fat stores to the appetite centre in the brain) but more research is needed.

Illness or physical injury can make it more difficult for people to control their weight and some medications can also affect appetite, fat distribution and activity levels, for example, Corticosteroids and some antidepressants and sedatives.

11 Yo-yo dieting ruins your metabolism

There is no evidence that yo-yo dieting systematically 'winds down' the metabolic rate, especially if you are overweight. But it can have a very detrimental effect on people's confidence in their ability to lose weight. This in itself can have a negative impact on future weight-loss success. However, short bouts of 'crash' dieting by people who are not initially overweight may cause a greater loss of muscle than is ideal and should be avoided.

12 There's no point exercising as it just increases my appetite

A number of studies show that regular exercise actually helps to regulate rather than increase appetite. It also has such a 'feel good' effect that it can encourage people to eat healthily in order to keep doing themselves some good. Regular exercise can also increase muscle mass, which in turn increases metabolic rate for as long as the extra muscle is maintained. In fact, a 1.4kg (3lb) increase in muscle mass can mean you burn enough extra calories to potentially lose 4.5kg (10lb) over a year. There is also a small and short-term boost in metabolic rate (for about 30 minutes) after a period of exercise has finished.

Now that you've read all the facts, complete this quiz before reading on.

(The quiz, written by Lyndel Costain, first appeared on www.malehealth.co.uk)

QUIZ DOES YOUR LIFESTYLE PUT YOU AT RISK OF BECOMING OBESE?

1 **What is your body mass index?** (see page 20)

18.5–24.9	0
25–29.9	2
30–34.9	4
35–39.9	6

Score:

2 **What is your waist measurement?** (see page 22)

For men

Less than 37in	0
37 to 39¾in	2
40in or more	4

For women

Less than 32in	0
32 to 34¾in	2
35in or more	4

Score:

3 **How many of your parents have had a weight problem?**

None	0
One	1
Both	2

Score:

4 **Physical activity**

Score 1 for each question you answer with NO.

a Do you usually walk up stairs rather than take the lift? YES/NO
b Do you walk briskly, or do some similar moderately intense activity, for 30 minutes on at least five days a week? YES/NO
c Do you spend much of the day on your feet? YES/NO
d Do you usually walk or cycle to the local shops or nearby places instead of driving? YES/NO
e Do you do something other than watch television most nights? YES/NO

Score:

5 **Eating habits**

Score 1 for each question you answer with YES.

a Do you often miss meals during the day and make up for it at night? YES/NO

b Do you regularly have second helpings? YES/NO

c Do you often eat for reasons other than hunger, e.g. if you are bored, angry or upset? YES/NO

d Do you eat chips, other fried foods or takeaways on at least four days a week? YES/NO

e Do you frequently snack on high-fat foods like crisps, pastries, cheese or chocolate? YES/NO

f Do you usually buy full-fat milk, dairy foods, spreads and oil-based dressings? YES/NO

g Do you regularly exceed healthy alcohol limits – 2–3 units a day for women and 3–4 a day (see page 81)? YES/NO

Score:

Now add all the scores together for your **FINAL SCORE**. How did you do?

0–8 Low risk – You're doing very well, keep it up!

9–14 Moderate risk – You may already be overweight, or even obese, but if not, your lifestyle puts you at risk of becoming so.

15–24 High risk – You will already be overweight or obese, or at high risk of becoming obese. Perhaps it is time to lose some pounds for your health's sake, or at least not gain any more.

section
2

the six-step guide

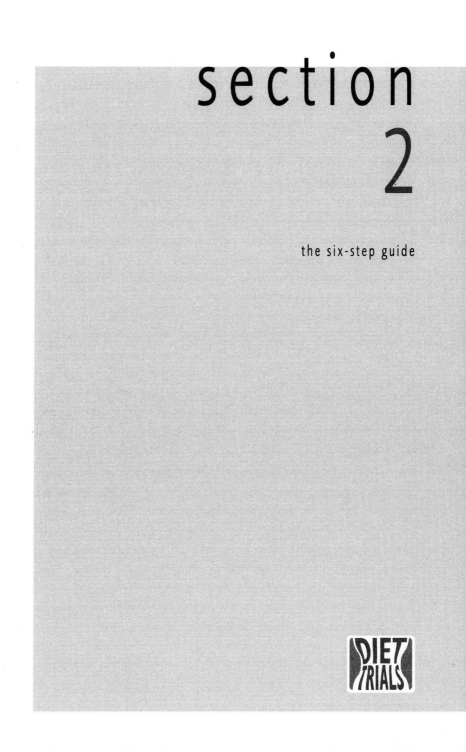

step one

WHY DO YOU WANT TO LOSE WEIGHT?

If you have got this far, you're obviously interested in losing some weight. You may have already assessed the healthiness of your weight using the guides in Section One. If you haven't why not do so now, remembering that the tools are a guide only. The important thing is to be a weight that is compatible with good health and that can be managed comfortably.

You have also probably realized that the *Diet Trials* is not yet another one-dimensional diet book, telling you what to do. Instead, it is a blueprint for assembling the pieces of the weight-control jigsaw that suit you best. It recognizes you as an individual. And will help you to become a motivated, skilled and confident problem-solver, making your own choices about the best way to survive the toxic environment.

To survive you must first plan your assault. A good place to start is to have a long hard think about why you want to lose weight, and what the consequences will be. In our 'slim is beautiful' culture, most people understandably want to lose weight to look better. This unfair pressure to conform to a certain size and shape has long been greater for women than for men, but today men are also subject to it – just look at the covers of men's health magazines and aftershave advertisements. Social pressures to conform to a slim ideal aren't right or fair, but they do exist. However, as you will have read in Section One, being overweight is really a health concern. *Diet Trials* will help you to address both issues. If you are a parent, it will also help you to be a good role model for your children. All this doesn't mean it's wrong to think that achieving a healthier weight will also help you to feel more self-confident and happier with your appearance.

Write down why you want to lose weight. Have a good think about all the possible benefits, for example: clothes will fit better; can play with son in the park; back will improve etc. Also think in terms of what you feel your weight is stopping you from doing now.

Health, Appearance and Self-Esteem

Psychologists have found that if people focus on appearance as their main reason to lose weight, they are less likely to succeed in the longterm. This seems to be because it doesn't raise their self-esteem (how they regard themselves). Instead their motivation to lose weight is spurred on by feeling bad about themselves; 'My fat looks disgusting, I must lose weight'; 'I hate myself for my lack of willpower.' If you start from a basis of feeling you are a lesser person because of your weight, and live in fear of being judged by your appearance, it's all so easy to fall at the first hurdle of change.

Identifying key motivations, for weight loss other than simply how you look – such as health and other aspects of physical and emotional well-being – is like saying that you're worth making changes for, and are actually a pretty OK person. It helps to boost your self-esteem before you even begin to lose weight. This is a very positive starting point because it allows you to view making changes to your diet and activity levels as good, even enjoyable things to do – not negative deprivations and hard work. Focus on what you want (being slimmer) not how fat you are, and expect to succeed.

ARE YOU REALLY READY TO LOSE WEIGHT?

You are still reading this book, and hopefully have thought carefully about why you want to lose weight. Now comes the next crunch. Are you really ready to do it? In other words, have you thought about the implications of your decision? If you have lost weight in the past, only, like so many, to put it all back on – have you thought about why that was? And how confident do you feel about being successful this time?

When you think of losing weight, you may think primarily about the weight you'd like to get to. However, weight loss only happens as a result of making changes to your usual eating and activity patterns. Making these changes is easier if you have a lot to gain; but there will also be associated costs. For example, overeating and extra weight actually benefits some people by helping them feel strong and assertive, or by stopping their partner getting jealous. So it helps enormously if you feel ready to work through the changes and choices needed to achieve your long-term goals.

'If you do what you've always done, you'll get what you've always got.'

A good starting point is to see how important making these changes is to you, and how confident you feel about making them.

So where would you place yourself on the following scales?

Importance

How important is it to you to make the changes that will allow you to lose weight?

0										10
Not at all important							Extremely important			

If you ranked yourself halfway or less along the scale, it might not be important enough for you to achieve the changes that will allow you to lose weight. If this is the case, have a rethink in a couple of weeks.

Confidence

How confident are you in your ability to make the changes that will allow you to lose weight?

|0 | | | | | | | | | 10|

Not at all confident   Extremely confident

Now ask yourself:

1 Why did I place myself at this point?
2 (If anything) what is stopping me moving further up the scale?
3 What things, people, support would help me to move further up?

QUIZ ARE YOU READY TO ACHIEVE A HEALTHIER WEIGHT?

Before you embark on your weight-control journey try this quiz just to see if you're starting off with the right attitude and outlook. It's all too easy to plunge in without considering your true needs and how you think and feel about food, as well as the situations or thoughts that have ruined your progress in the past.

Answer TRUE or FALSE to the following statements.

1 My goal is to lose a lot of weight. Only then will I be happy with my weight.
2 I accept the wisdom that it's best to lose weight gradually.
3 I have spent time thinking about my current lifestyle, for example, my eating habits and how active I am.
4 I now realize that to be successful I need permanent, not temporary, changes to the way I eat and how physically active I am.
5 I'm thinking of losing weight now because it is important to me, not for somebody else.
6 Losing weight will help me to deal with other problems in my life.
7 I am prepared to be more active on a regular basis.

8   I can only lose weight successfully if I don't break my diet.

9   I realize that to lose weight and keep it off means that I will need to spend some time learning more about food and ways to be more active, and plan ahead each week to help me make changes to the way I currently eat, and how active I am.

10 My main motivation for losing weight is because I loathe how I look.

Now work out your score

Give yourself one point if you answered TRUE to questions 2, 3, 4, 5, 7 and 9. Give yourself one point for answering FALSE to questions 1, 6, 8 and 10. Any score over 7 indicates that you have a positive and realistic approach to weight controls, and are more likely to succeed long-term. If you scored less than 4, probably, it is not a good time to start until you've had a rethink! Your answers also reflect potential stumbling blocks to achieving your weight loss goals. [Adapted with permission, from the 'Weight Loss Readiness Quiz' (American Dietetic Association)]

What are the Pros and Cons of Lifestyle Changes?

When you make a choice to change something, it will have an impact on other things. If you start to lose weight without fully appreciating this it can throw you off course or make you give up altogether. But being aware of the possible pros and cons can help you feel less frustrated over potential conflicts. This also boosts your motivation and the belief that you have made the right choices.

Weigh up the pros and cons of the lifestyle changes required to lose weight. Write them down (see example opposite). If you decide that the pros outweigh the cons, then great. If you find it's the other way round, this may not be the best time to lose weight. If you are still unsure then why not try the goal-setting approach in Step Three, for a couple of weeks? Use that experience to decide whether you want to continue, or come back to losing weight some time in the future.

Making lifestyle changes now

Pros – For	Cons – Against
Feeling more energetic	Have to put in time, thought
Feeling slimmer in clothes	and energy

Not making lifestyle changes – how would I feel in 6 months' time?

Pros – For	Cons – Against
Didn't have to worry	My bad back and breathlessness
about failing	will probably be worse

SKILLS FOR SLIMMING SUCCESS

It's Not About Willpower!

Willpower isn't really something you have or you don't have. Willpower – or what seems like it – is a skill. It's a sign that you've made a conscious choice to do something, based on your thoughts about the consequences of that choice or action. For example, the person who would love to party with their friends but instead stays in to finish an important report could be said to have 'strong willpower'. What has really happened is that they have made the choice to work since the consequences are that they're more likely to finish something that will help shape their future. There was some pain, but the potential pay-off was high.

Everything we do is preceded by a thought. Very often it doesn't seem like it because things can happen automatically. Just one 'will-full thought' can be enough to get us through short-term events, like studying for an exam or staying off the booze on a Friday night before a sporting game! You may also be able to survive a short strict diet. But your basic hunger drive, the toxic environment and your lack of coping skills will soon overwhelm you, the diet will be 'broken' and the weight will come back on. And while you might have lost some weight for a short time, you have not achieved your real goal of reaching and maintaining a healthier weight. Changing your eating and activity behaviours are things that you have to stay conscious of over the longterm; they can't be sustained by simply 'willing' them to happen.

Skills

Learning new skills is the key to successful weight control. And the real trick is working out how to use these skills to make lifestyle changes that are relevant to your needs.

You might still think you don't need skills, just 'willpower' or 'a good telling off' to make you lose weight. But there's only so long that you, or somebody else, can hit you over the head to 'make' you do something. Your head, and your self-confidence, will soon suffer. And our toxic environment, with its bewildering array of food choices, labour-saving devices, confusing diets, stresses and time pressures constantly throws up new scenarios that we have to get to grips with.

Or it may be that you have such a low opinion of yourself that you sabotage your weight loss attempts because you don't feel you're worth the care and effort. Perhaps you aren't assertive enough to say 'no' to food, even if you don't want it. Or maybe, despite being desperate to lose weight, you define yourself as 'not being able to cope if you can't eat what you want, when you want'. In this case you would benefit from changing your attitude and 'self-definition'.

All these scenarios would benefit from skills – and skills need practice. Think in terms of, say, learning to play the piano. You don't just expect to be able to play it. You have to learn and reinforce new skills such as reading music and learning new pieces. If you don't play for a while your technique will get rusty, and you may even be tempted to give up altogether. So you need to plan ways to ensure you keep up your practice and stay on track. When it comes to weight loss, developing the skills of thinking ahead, setting achievable personal goals, planning your days around them and learning how to cope when things don't go to plan, will give you the confidence to make the changes you want.

STRATEGIES OF SUCCESSFUL SLIMMERS

Get ready to be inspired! There's nothing quite like success stories to boost confidence and self-belief in what you can achieve. Not surprisingly, those who do succeed view their weight as something they can manage rather than something they have no control over. Phrases like 'I just have to look at food and I put on weight' or 'I will never be slim as I simply can't resist chocolate' no longer pass their lips. Some people seem to have these skills naturally, others get this 'control' by working out changes for themselves – rather than following rigid plans. In other words, successful slimmers are usually those who glean useful information from a variety of sources and use it to develop their own healthy weight-loss strategies.

There have been some outstanding research studies that examine exactly what successful slimmers do – and how their strategies differ from those of people who regain their lost weight.One heartening survey of 20,000 readers of a magazine in the US found that 72 per cent of people who had lost weight (an average of 15kg/34lb) and kept it off, had ultimately done it on their own, compared to only 20 per cent in commercial slimming groups.

One big question, of course, is 'How is success measured?' This is where setting personal and achievable goals comes into play (see Step Two). And now that we know that a 10 per cent weight loss brings big health benefits, this – rather than getting right down to a usually unachievable 'slim' weight – has become a new measure of success.

The first study to look at 'slimming success' was published in the *American Journal of Clinical Nutrition*, back in 1990. But its findings are still incredibly relevant today. Three specific groups of women were questioned: maintainers (lost weight then stayed at their goal weight for at least two years); relapsers (lost and regained their excess weight a number of times) and controls (had always been a healthy weight). The key findings were:

Weight-loss methods

Most maintainers

- Used classic weight-loss strategies such as being more active, eating more healthily and having smaller portions, and devised ways to fit these strategies into their lives – rather than follow rigid diets.
- Reported that they were patient about their progress, setting small goals they could meet, and 'sticking to' plans they had devised personally (taking information from a variety of sources) until new habits were established.
- Ate regular meals and few snacks.
- Found that they eventually did not want to eat as much, and that very fatty and sweet foods lost their regular appeal. They switched to lower-fat cooking methods and ate more fruit and vegetables.
- Found that food became less important in their lives. They had no 'forbidden' ones and occasionally ate small amounts of their favourite foods which helped avoid feelings of deprivation i.e. 'flexible restraint' (see page 147).
- Confronted problems directly rather than avoiding them or using food.
- Used support from others, such as family, friends or health professionals.

Most relapsers

- Did not exercise to lose weight.
- Followed or took formula diets or appetite suppressants, fasted, or followed rigid diet plans or programmes they couldn't sustain.
- Skipped breakfast and ate more snacks, especially confectionery.
- Felt deprived most of the time. They banned their favourite (high-fat)

foods and viewed their diet foods as different to what they really wanted to eat, and what the family could eat.

- Regained weight in response to a negative life event that interfered with their access to their 'diet foods'.
- Ate unconsciously in response to emotions and did not confront problems directly.
- Didn't use or seek support from others, such as family, friends or health professionals.

Diets tried in the past

If you have tried losing weight before it can help to look back and see what your experiences were. You may find that even though they didn't help overall, you found some things that could be useful pieces in your personal weight-management jigsaw. For example, although you found that a slimming group wasn't for you, you did find sharing things with others helpful and now make sure you ask someone to support you. Make some notes to help you learn from your personal dieting history, for example:

Diet/programme	Outcome	What was helpful	What was unhelpful
Grapefruit diet	Lost 4lb but only lasted 6 days	Decided never to try a crash diet again	Rigid and impractical food restrictions

STARTING A FOOD DIARY

One skill that is vital for long-term success is 'self-monitoring' – a record that assesses and tracks how, what, when and why you eat, and how active you are. It is a key technique of a psychological approach called 'cognitive behavioural therapy' (CBT). Because scientific evidence supports this therapy as being one of the best ways to help people control their weight, most of the guidance in this book is based on CBT approaches. These will help you develop the skills to identify and change unhelpful thoughts, behaviours and feelings that get in the way of you making lifestyle changes that lead to slimming success. People often think that keeping a diary or record is unnecessary or too time consuming. Or they may even find the idea of writing down everything they eat a bit embarrassing! But it really is worth doing. The bottom line is: people who *do* self-monitor, *do* lose weight.

Getting Started

The simplest way to start a food diary is to write down absolutely everything you eat and drink over the day. Use a handy-sized notebook you can carry with you and record things as you go along rather than trying to remember it all at the end of the day. Write down when you are eating, and also where you are. At this stage, try not to change your normal eating patterns. This record is your baseline to build from. Also make a note of any activity during the day that lasts for at least 10 minutes. Keep the diary up for a full week, or longer if you like, before you start using it to plan changes. Some people like to write down their thoughts and/or make a note of how hungry they were when they ate. This is especially helpful for people who often eat when they aren't physically hungry, but for other reasons. (If that sounds like you, read the section on 'Head Hunger' on page 136 before you start your diary.)

Writing down everything you eat and drink can be difficult, so don't expect to be an instant expert. Like all new skills it takes practice. Use the diary as a constructive tool that will help you to recognize, change and review problem areas and negative thoughts – rather than something to tell yourself off about. The more honest you can be with yourself, the more you will be helped. It's the little things that make the difference.

SAMPLE FOOD AND ACTIVITY DIARY

This is an example of the kind of information that can be useful for you to record when you start keeping a diary. Make sure you write down absolutely everything that passes your lips.

Date *Wednesday 5 August*

Time	Food and drink	Where/who with	Comments
8 a.m.	Coffee with s/s milk	At home, with partner	Rushing to work
9 a.m.	Chocolate croissant Cappuccino	Coffee shop near work alone	Just a habit
1 p.m.	Tuna sandwich, crisps	At desk	Busy, just ate it
3 p.m.	Chocolate bar, coffee	At desk	Needed sugar – felt stressed at work
5 p.m.	Few biscuits, coffee	At work	Needed food before the pub
6 p.m.	3 large wines. crisps	At pub with colleague	
9 p.m.	Chicken korma, 1 naan, pilau rice, 2 poppadoms	At home with partner	Hungry, no food in fridge but now feel stuffed full

Activity – Walked to and from home to train to work (detour for pub) – 30 minutes in total

step two

setting smart goals

Imagine that your big dream is to be a champion showjumper, even though you don't know how to ride. Achieving it will change your life. All you need is determination. You would be happy and admired.

Suddenly, you have the time and opportunity to learn. But now that it's become a reality, you realize you can no longer expect to get on the horse and head for the Olympics. You revise your goals and take things a step a time. Being a showjumper, let alone a champion, is expecting too much and trying to achieve it would dominate your life. You decide that simply learning to ride and jump, and the personal satisfaction this will bring, is plenty. It will be achievable and something you can keep up. Your decision bolsters your belief in your abilities to succeed.

First you need to learn how to ride a horse. Then, as your confidence grows, feel your way with the jumps. And if you fall off at one of the first hurdles, you or others won't say 'Oh dear, you had your chance and you failed, so you should give up.' You will pick yourself up, remind yourself of all the important reasons why you are doing this, get back on the horse, refocus on your goals, reinforce the skills you feel comfortable with, and move on – won't you?

If you agree with the theme of this story, I wonder if you would feel the same if it was changed – and was about you and weight loss. If, for example, the big dream was that you would get down from a size 18 (and rising) to a size 10, a size you had never been before. A size you felt would free you from being fat and out of control – and change your life. A size that you should be able to get to with willpower. Sadly, a size that you don't achieve because your goals are unrealistic, and your diet plan is too strict to follow for long – and makes you fall at the first hurdle!

Does this second scenario sound familiar? If so, can you see how the two stories are actually quite similar to start with, but the first takes a logical change for the better? Can you see how valid this approach would be for long-term weight-loss success? How falling at the first or second hurdle doesn't mean you have ruined everything and so must give up? Instead, it is all part of the learning experience. How setting realistic and maintainable goals, and acquiring the skills and confidence to achieve them, might just mean that you actually realize more than a dream? In the case of the second scenario this could be feeling healthy, attractive, sociable, in control – and being a wonderful size 14.

WHAT SHOULD YOUR GOAL WEIGHT BE?

There is no single answer to the question of what a person's goal weight should be. As discussed in Section One, there isn't an 'ideal' weight for anyone. Even official guides, such as the BMI, used for assessing the healthiness of weight are about weight or waist 'ranges', rather than single numbers. And it could well be that actually getting into a healthy weight range isn't realistic nor necessary. In Section One we also talked about the benefit of modest weight loss, and how losing just 5 to 10 per cent of your weight tends to be more sustainable and significantly benefits health.

This concept of not aiming to be as slim as possible can be tricky to get to grips with, since there is so much social pressure to conform to 'slim' or 'lean and muscular' ideals. But most of the research about long-term weight-loss success suggests that being realistic about weight-loss goals – and believing you are an OK person regardless of your weight – are a fundamental part of that success. It's easy to fall into the trap of measuring success in terms of how close you get to that 'dream weight', rather than how much weight you have actually lost and the benefits this brings. Being realistic means you are more likely to meet your expectations and so feel, and be, successful long term.

The research also suggests that, on average, most people don't keep off more than 10 per cent of their weight. This might seem alarming. But don't forget that you are still living in the toxic environment, and the fact that you are struggling with your weight may mean that you are genetically more susceptible than others to its effects. Just to stop gaining weight, let alone maintaining a healthy weight loss, is a fantastic achievement. And, of course, some people do lose and keep off more than this 10 per cent figure.

Back to the initial question of goal weights. Health experts working for the UK charity Weight Concern believe that, because we are all individual shapes and sizes, rather than focus on a weight to get to it's more helpful to learn to make lifestyle changes and accept whatever weight these changes lead to. In other words, aim to be a weight that's healthy and comfortable for you to maintain – rather than a weight dictated by fashion gurus.

There can, of course, be exceptions to every rule. If you are very overweight, you may find you have the skills to comfortably lose much more than 10 per cent of your weight – and maintain that loss. Or you may have a health problem that will only benefit adequately from a particular level of medically advised weight loss. In this case, weight loss (and the dietary and activity changes that enable you to achieve it) is actually part of the treatment for the condition, and is at least as important as any medication (see page 210).

Use the guides in Section One to help you get a feel for where your weight lies on the 'healthiness' scale. If you are above the healthy weight range, and decide you want to have a target, consider a first target of a 5 per cent loss. For example, if you weigh 89kg (14 stone) this would translate to a 4.5kg loss to reach 84.5kg (13 stone 4lb). Weigh yourself once or twice a week, preferably on the same day and at the same time (first thing in the morning is best). If you prefer not to think about numbers on the bathroom scales, you can track your waist size, how you fit into a certain item of clothing, or how your body composition or other body measurements change. Or you may like to combine some of these.

When considering goal weights or waist sizes, bear in mind any health problems you know you have. If you aren't sure about this, have a BMI of 35 or more, or think you are at risk of some of the health problems mentioned in this book, do have a chat with your doctor.

HOW TO SET SMART GOALS

'Old habits cannot be thrown out the upstairs window. They must be coaxed down the stairs one step at a time.' Mark Twain

There are no simple or magical solutions to long-term weight loss. And you can get frustrated – and fat – trying to find one. Despite what charlatans might tell you, losing weight requires motivation, skill and focus. But you will reap the rewards if you stay focused on what you want, trust your abilities and hone things to suit your needs. Planning and making changes that are achievable and sustainable is what works. Realistic goals enable you to acquire knowledge, develop the necessary skills and so stay confident and motivated. Most importantly, they build self-esteem and belief in your own abilities (otherwise known as 'self-efficacy').

They are the backbone of your long-term slimming success. They swell confidence in your ability to manage change, rather than making you fall at the first or second hurdle, feel a failure and give up. A simple way to give your goals a reality check is to see if they are SMART – Specific, Measurable, Achievable, Relevant and/or Time-specific.

For example, you may eat chocolate at least once a day, and see it as one of your key problems. So you set yourself a goal of 'giving up chocolate'. You might be able to achieve this for a while, but it's impossible to sustain. Eventually you eat some chocolate, think you've broken your diet and probably keep on eating chocolate – then abandon everything. Instead you could set a SMART goal of 'having chocolate twice a week for the next two weeks, and have fruit for snacks on the other days. If it goes well, you can renew the goal.

SMART stands for

S – Specific

If your goal is 'to eat more healthily', that is very general. You could start with a specific goal so that you know exactly what you want to do: 'From tomorrow I will aim to have breakfast cereal topped with fruit every morning, and at least two vegetables with my evening meal.'

M – Measurable

You may set a measurable goal of having, for example, at least five portions of fruit and vegetables each day. You could tick each portion off on a checklist as you go.

A – Achievable

Make sure your goal is realistic. Staying with the fruit and vegetable example, if you normally struggle to eat one or two portions five could be ambitious, and three would be more achievable. You can then plan small steps towards achieving this – for example, have juice with breakfast, take fruit to work for snacks. Once you get used to three portions, you could aim for the recommended five a day.

R – Relevant

Choose a goal that is important and relevant to your true needs, rather than a goal you (or others) feel you should have. For example, if you have already reduced your fat intake, but skip meals a lot, having regular meals would be a more important goal than say, switching from semi-skimmed to skimmed milk.

T – Time-specific

Give yourself a realistic timescale to achieve your goal – this is likely to be weeks rather than days. If things go well, you can renew the time period. Changing the habits of a lifetime has its ups and downs, and doesn't happen overnight. Also, when setting a new goal a time limit can be used to help you to 'experiment' to see if it's right for you, rather than committing yourself to something you find you can't manage – with the result that you feel a failure and abandon things altogether.

Here are some more examples of how you can turn general goals into SMART goals. Whenever you plan goals, see how they measure up to the SMART principles.

General goal:

Easter eggs are my downfall so I won't eat any this year.

SMART goal:

I will ask people at work not to buy me Easter eggs this year. Instead I will enjoy just a couple of small, specially nice ones rather than eat loads. I could also suggest to friends and family that they buy me some nice flowers instead of chocolate.

General goal:

After the festive celebrations I feel I should lose a stone in January.

SMART goal:

I will cut right down on all the high-fat snacking I was doing thanks to festive fare, and do 30 minutes of walking most days throughout January. This will help me lose some weight slowly and steadily.

SETTING YOUR OWN SMART GOALS

Once you embark on making lifestyle changes goal-setting will be a really important skill. This book will give you two approaches to change. One is about assessing your problem areas and making changes to your current eating and activity habits. The other is a more structured eating plan combined with regular physical activity. Both will involve goal-setting, food diaries and other elements of cognitive behavioural therapy (see page 54) to help you develop your own strategies for managing your weight. Have a look at the guide to SMART goal-setting on the following page. It helps you to decide how you will achieve small goals that will lead to your overall goal of weight loss. Plan to reward yourself for achieving each goal – preferably with something that doesn't involve food, like a trip to the cinema, a new magazine, whatever!

Start date:

Goal
E.g. Take lunch to work each day to avoid high-fat meals in the canteen.

Date to check progress:

Things I will do to achieve my goal
E.g. Plan my shopping ahead so that I have ingredients for a healthy packed lunch; make sure I have 5 minutes to spare in the morning to make sandwiches; make use of the fridge at work.

How achieving this goal will help me
E.g. It will stop me buying high-fat cooked lunches or mayonnaise-ridden sandwiches and being tempted by desserts as I wait in the queue to pay. Will help me save some money too.

What barriers might get in the way?
E.g. Not having the right food in the house or not leaving enough time to make lunch; colleagues complain that I am being boring; can't resist old favourites on the canteen menu.

How will I deal with them?
E.g. Plan what I will have when I do the main shopping; make my sandwiches the night before and freeze them if need be; tell my colleagues that making this change is very important to me; occasionally – once or twice a fortnight – have a true favourite when it's on the menu, and really enjoy it.

What I will reward myself with when I achieve it by my review date
E.g. Go and see a new-release film.

step three

part one

FOOD – MAKING THE MOST OF IT

If you're still reading you're probably still interested in losing weight, or maybe simply in maintaining your weight and eating better. If you do want to lose weight, hopefully you've thought about why and realized that quick-fix diets aren't the answer. Believing in your abilities and setting personal goals for achievable and sustainable changes are the keys to long-term slimming success.

Maybe this is the first part of *Diet Trials* you've turned to, because you want to see what its diet plan will let you eat! If so, by all means have a look. However, you'll probably find that you need to read the earlier parts of the book first to see how the following skills and information about food and nutrition will help you best.

Like this Step, Steps Four and Five are also very practical, and there is no correct order for reading any of these Steps. If you feel you binge or comfort eat a lot, or think you're a bit of a yo-yo dieter, it may help to read Step Four first. If you are really interested in activity, then read Step Five. The choice is yours!

Back to food. This Step will provide a lot of information about a healthy diet and, hopefully, the opportunity to learn new skills about food choice and preparation, balanced meals and eating styles. With the vast amount and variety of food now available, knowing how to choose and enjoy a healthy diet really is fundamental to surviving the toxic environment and, as a result, managing your weight in the long term. It will also benefit your general health and well-being.

You may already know quite a bit about food – we all have to eat, and many of us provide meals for our families – but do take the time to read all this Step, not just the meal planners. Even if it largely reinforces what you already know you should still find it helpful. There is a lot of poor advice around about food, health and weight, which is not based on good nutritional science, and *Diet Trials* will hopefully set the record straight. Once again, 'knowledge is power'. This Step also gives up-to-date advice on the sort of diet that best helps weight control, as well as guidance on how to manage the amount you eat flexibly, in order to take in less calories than you burn and so gradually lose weight.

WHAT IS A HEALTHY DIET?

With the number of newspaper headlines dedicated to the latest 'diet discovery', or debates about whether butter is better than margarine or wheat is bad for you, you may well wonder what you should be eating! While it might seem that the experts never agree, the good news is that there is widespread international consensus on what makes up a healthy diet. What you read or hear in the media is usually the result of just one study or comments from self-styled 'experts' who express personal beliefs rather than science. And even science must be thoroughly reviewed before dietary recommendations are made.

Of course, all forms of science constantly evolve as new evidence emerges from good quality research. Nutritional science is no exception, which means there's always some fine-tuning going on. For example, it is healthy to have carbohydrate-rich foods as part of a meal, but we now know that some are better choices than others because of the rate at which they are digested and absorbed.

National food guides have been developed by different countries to give guidance on what makes up a healthy and balanced diet. The American guide is shaped as a food pyramid, while in the UK a plate-shaped guide called the 'Balance of Good Health' is used.

The 'Balance of Good Health' is literally about balance and variety rather than which foods are 'good' or 'bad'. All foods are 'legal' in a healthy diet, and the same goes when you are eating to lose weight. It is true that many of us could do with eating more fruit and vegetables and cutting back on fatty and sugary foods – not to mention big portions. But the emphasis is really on enjoying more of the foods that protect and nourish our bodies, and optimize health. In other words, how we can make the most of food.

Balanced Eating Basics

- Enjoy a variety of foods from each of the five food segments every day, as outlined in the 'Balance of Good Health' on page 67.
- Each segment represents one of the five main food groups that make up a balanced diet. The size of the segments varies according to the healthiest proportions for each group – this is why the fruit and vegetable segment is the largest, and the fatty and sugary is the smallest.
- Foods in each group are good sources of similar nutrients, so can be interchanged to add variety and meet individual food and diet preferences – for example, those of vegetarians.
- By following the guidelines you will automatically choose a diet built on a base of vegetables, fruit and energy-giving carbohydrates. It will also be moderate in protein but low in saturated fat, and brimming with vital vitamins, minerals and antioxidants.
- The 'Balance of Good Health' is designed for adults of all ages and for children from five years of age. (Young children, pregnant and breastfeeding women, and people with medical conditions requiring special diets, have more specific needs.)

How Does a Healthy Diet Benefit Our Health?

If you are going to make changes of any type it's always good to know what the benefits are, to help you stay motivated. Changing your diet is no exception, as it is such an important part of day-to-day life. Here are just some of the reasons why a healthy diet is good for all of us. It might be worth making a list of your own reasons for eating more healthily too.

In the shorter term a healthy diet:

- Is vital for children's growth and development.
- Maintains healthy hair, eyes and nails and a regular bowel.
- Gives you the energy for day-to-day living, and for exercise.
- Helps memory, mood and concentration.
- Helps you to stay in shape.
- Helps you to fight infections and recover more quickly from illness.

In the longer term a healthy diet:

- Reduces the risk of health problems such as obesity, diabetes, heart disease, various cancers, high blood pressure, stroke, cataracts, depression and osteoporosis (brittle bones).
- Helps you to stay fit and healthy as you get older.

What Can Get In the Way of Eating More Healthily?

We choose to eat certain foods for lots of different reasons. Taste is the biggest decider, but cost, health, convenience, tradition, food availability, social influences, hunger, emotions, peer-pressure and pure pleasure are some of the many others. It's no wonder then, that changing our eating habits is not a straightforward process. And it affects not only you but also others close to you.

Because we live in a society where there is plenty of food, what and why we eat is very much influenced by habit or automatic learned responses, which have nothing to do with true physical hunger. For example, we may like to relax in front of the television after a hard day at work, with a drink and something to munch on. Before long,

The balance of good health

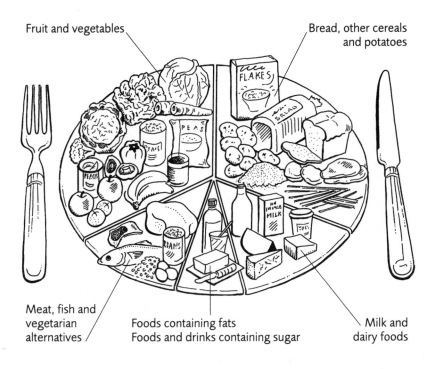

Fruit and vegetables

Bread, other cereals and potatoes

Meat, fish and vegetarian alternatives

Foods containing fats
Foods and drinks containing sugar

Milk and dairy foods

watching television at any time could become a trigger to eat something. Feeling angry or insecure are other common triggers, especially if you find it hard to express your emotions. Food can serve as a useful means of stuffing that anger or insecurity back down. And before long eating becomes a habit, so automatic that it often feels as though you're out of control around food, and you simply can't get a healthier balance to your diet.

For some, a barrier to changing to a healthier diet can be the fear that this will mean having to give up favourite foods. Or it could be too time consuming, or you will have to eat differently from the rest of the family, or from your friends. Not wanting to miss out on social events, meals out or holiday fun can be other barriers. Having the confidence to say 'no' to people offering you food can also be hard.

Maybe more practical issues – the cost or even the taste of healthier food, not knowing what foods to choose, lack of healthy choices at work or when eating away from home – are barriers. Or it may be that so many diet books you have read in the past have told you to 'avoid that', 'eat this freely', 'combine this with that' and 'under no circumstances eat once it's dark' that you are understandably confused by food rules!

If you want to change how you eat, but find there are too many barriers to keep your good intentions up, why not write them down now. Even though some might seem almost insurmountable, there is always a way around them. Have a think and write down how you may overcome them. Successful slimmers do it all the time.

For example, a barrier could be:
'I don't like vegetables or other healthy food very much.'

And a positive way round it:
'I could overcome this by experimenting with different foods and vegetables and learning to cook them in different ways, like stir-fries, in curries or pasta sauces. A healthy cookbook would be helpful too.'

The Diet-Overeat Cycle

Another barrier can come from yo-yo dieting with quick-fix diets. You get so stuck on the diet cycle that you rarely get time to reap the benefits of eating healthily because you are busy lurching from one set of diet rules to the next – with some hefty comfort-eating in between!

As you will see from the diagram on page 70, this self-destructive cycle does nothing for your self-esteem and self-efficacy (belief in your own abilities). If it looks familiar, check out ways to help break free in Step Four.

CHOOSING A HEALTHY DIET

Now for the low-down on the different food groups that make up a healthy diet and how you can change the quality of your diet for the better. It will really help if you can compare the following recommendations with how you are eating now. If you aren't yet keeping a daily food diary (see page 52), keep one for a few days so that you have some record for comparison.

Using the portion guides for each of the following food groups, decide on approximately how many portions you currently eat. Don't worry if your diet is way out of whack – you won't be alone! The toxic environment can make it hard to eat healthily unless you consciously choose to do so. Then, with skills and practice, it becomes a natural and thoroughly enjoyable habit.

This is general advice only, so if you have specific questions about keeping your, or your family's, diet balanced, ask your doctor to refer you to the practice nurse, local health visitor or state-registered dietitian. At this stage, the healthy eating advice isn't specifically about how to lose weight; it is mainly intended to improve the balance and quality of your day-to-day food choices.

BREADS, POTATOES, RICE, CEREALS, PASTA AND GRAINS

Key nutrients: Carbohydrate (mainly starchy), fibre, B vitamins including folic acid, potassium, iron, magnesium, selenium, some protein, essential fats, calcium and vitamin E. Phytochemicals.

These foods are packed with healthy energy (and the B vitamins needed to release energy from food) and are naturally low in fat, so it is sensible to make them part of every meal. Good choices include different types of bread, breakfast cereals, oats, pasta, potatoes, noodles and rice or other grains.

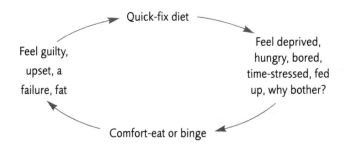

Quick-fix diet

Feel guilty, upset, a failure, fat

Feel deprived, hungry, bored, time-stressed, fed up, why bother?

Comfort-eat or binge

Aim to include some whole-grain varieties each day, such as wholemeal bread, porridge, bran flakes, Shredded Wheat, Weetabix, brown rice, rye crispbread, wholewheat pasta or popcorn. If you don't like wholemeal bread, try granary bread or whole grain cereals. Whole grains add more fibre to the diet (see page 86) and studies suggest that they help to reduce the risk of heart disease, certain cancers and type 2 diabetes by up to 30 per cent. They also help to keep you regular. Ideally, aim for three portions of whole-grain foods each day.

Some breads and breakfast cereals are fortified with extra nutrients like iron, folic acid and other B vitamins, and make especially good choices when you are slimming, or for children and teenage girls who are at most risk of lacking iron in their diet.

If you need to avoid wheat or gluten (a protein found in wheat, barley, rye and possibly oats) for medical reasons* keep your diet balanced with other grains such as rice, millet, buckwheat, sago, quinoa or sweetcorn as well as breads, pasta and other foods made from gluten-free grains.

* Check any suspected wheat or gluten intolerance with your doctor. It could be due to coeliac disease, a lifelong condition that needs a strict diet and medical attention. If left untreated, it could have serious health effects.

Aim to have 5–11 portions daily (according to your appetite and calorie needs). A portion could be:

- A slice of bread
- 3 tablespoons breakfast cereal

- Half a bagel, half a pitta bread or half an English muffin
- 3 crackers or rice cakes
- 2 rounded tablespoons cooked rice
- 3 rounded tablespoons pasta or noodles
- 1 medium potato

HOW MANY DAILY PORTIONS DO YOU CURRENTLY HAVE? ____

HOW MANY OF THESE ARE WHOLEGRAIN? ____

Can I afford to eat more healthily?

Some people have less money to spend on food than others and feel this is a big barrier. If this is true for you, don't feel that you can't make any changes. Whenever anybody sets realistic goals, they will be realistic for their needs and circumstances. This book suggests lots of possible changes, so start with the ones that are most manageable and affordable. Planning ahead and shopping differently will help. For example, it usually costs less to buy fruit and veg in a street market rather than from a supermarket, and frozen and canned produce can be cheaper than fresh ones. Cutting right back on fatty and sugary snacks foods, and preparing meals at home in place of high-fat takeaways will save money. See page 120 for advice on how to adapt family meals without having to spend more.

Make the most of breads, other cereals and potatoes

- Try different breads and find tasty ones that don't need extra spread.
- If you fancy some chips occasionally, opt for low-fat oven chips or thick-cut potato wedges.
- Leave the skins on new and jacket potatoes, and try sweet potatoes for a change – they are even more nutritious.
- Experiment with the unique flavours of different types of rice –

Basmati, jasmine, wild, red, brown or Arborio to mention a few.

- Vary your types of noodles and pasta, too, and include those made from rice, corn or buckwheat.
- Choose steamed or boiled rice or noodles rather than fried.
- Top pasta with vegetable or tomato-based sauces rather than creamy or cheesy ones.
- Serve breakfast cereals with chilled skimmed or semi-skimmed milk and go for whole grain types. (Watch crunchy oat cereals – they're loaded with fat and sugar.)
- Breakfast cereals can make quick, low fat snacks any time of the day – just limit your portion size.

FRUIT AND VEGETABLES

Key nutrients Vitamin C, folic acid, beta-carotene, fibre, magnesium, potassium, some carbohydrate, iron and calcium. Phytochemicals.

Most of us could benefit from eating more fruit and vegetables. Not only do they add colour and texture to meals, they are filling, low calorie and help to reduce the risk of developing health problems such as heart disease, cancers, obesity and cataracts. They even seem to help to keep our bones strong and lungs healthy. Studies suggest that the benefits are greatest if we eat at least five portions of a variety of fruit and vegetables each day. Some experts recommend nine a day!

Nutritionist scientists have finally worked out 'why' mum was – and still is – right to tell us to 'eat our greens'. It's the vitamins, minerals, fibre and protective phytochemicals and antioxidants in fruit and vegetables that make them so good for us.

Different coloured fruit and vegetables reflect the presence of different phytochemicals (natural plant compounds), so vary them for the optimal health-protecting mix. And if fitting in five or more portions sounds difficult, take it step by step (don't forget SMART goals) and

Phytochemicals These are natural plant compounds (*phyto* = plant) found in fruit, vegetables, whole grains, nuts and seeds and they give plants their distinctive taste and colour. They seem to protect our health in different ways and help explain why these foods are so good for us. Some phytochemicals block the development of cancer cells, others influence chemical reactions that regulate body functions and many are antioxidants.

Antioxidants These work to mop up excess 'free radicals', highly reactive molecules that are by-products of basic bodily processes such as breathing and burning the energy in food. Free radicals are also increased by environmental stresses such as pollution, smoking and too much sun. They whiz around the body with the potential to damage healthy cells. If left unchecked by antioxidants, this cell damage may increase the risk of a wide range of health problems including heart disease, cancers, cataracts, lung problems and skin damage, and speed up the ageing process.

remember that fresh, frozen, canned, dried and juiced fruit and vegetables can all count.

Aim to have at least 5 portions every day. A portion (about 80g/3oz) could be:

- 2 tablespoons vegetables – fresh, frozen or canned (excluding potatoes)
- Dessert bowlful of salad
- Medium piece of fruit, e.g. orange, apple, banana
- 2 small fruit e.g., satsumas, plums
- Large slice of a large fruit, e.g. pineapple, melon
- 1 tablespoon dried fruit
- 3 tablespoons stewed or canned fruit
- Small glass of pure fruit juice (count this just once towards your 5 a day)

HOW MANY DAILY PORTIONS DO YOU CURRENTLY HAVE? _____

VITAMIN/ MINERAL	RNI (Reference Nutrient Intake)	WHAT IT DOES	WHERE IT'S FOUND
Vitamin A	600mcg for women 700mcg for men	Helps keep the skin, eyes and immune system healthy. Helps us see in the dark by protecting against night blindness.	Fish roe, liver, cheese, eggs, oily fish, butter and margarine. The body also converts beta-carotene found in green, orange and red vegetables and fruits, to vitamin A. Note that pregnant women should avoid liver and pâté as it is extremely rich in vitamin A, which may harm the developing baby.
Vitamin B_{12}	1.5mcg	Needed to form red blood cells and protect against macrocytic anaemia, and helps maintain the health of the nervous system and bone marrow.	Liver, kidney, meat, poultry, fish, dairy foods, eggs, B_{12} fortified foods such as soya milk, cereals and yeast extracts. Note that B_{12} is only naturally found in foods of animal origin so vegans need a regular intake of fortified foods.
Folic Acid	200mcg	A type of B vitamin that reduces the risk of spina bifida during pregnancy, works with B_{12} to reduce risk of heart disease. Also needed for healthy red blood cells, mood and nerve function.	Pulses, green leafy vegetables, yeast extracts, liver, orange juice, fortified cereals, nuts, avocados, lettuce.
Other B Vitamins		Let the body release and use energy from food. Help keep the skin, hair, eyes, nervous and digestive systems healthy.	Meat, fish, poultry, dairy foods, whole grains, eggs, nuts, seeds, pulses, green vegetables, fortified cereals and yeast extracts.
Vitamin C	40mg	A protective antioxidant needed for healthy skin, bones, teeth, gums and blood vessels, helps fight infection and boost iron absorption from non-meat foods.	Most fruit, vegetables and juices, but especially citrus fruits and juices, kiwi fruit, berries, blackcurrants, papaya, guava, peppers, green vegetables, peas and potatoes.
Vitamin D	None, since most comes from the action of sunlight on the skin	Needed for the body to absorb and use calcium to build and maintain strong bones. Aids immunity and might help to protect against cancer.	Most of our needs are met when vitamin D is generated by the action of some sunlight on the skin. An average of 20 to 30 minutes gentle exposure a day during spring and summer provides enough for the year (avoid sunburn). Food sources include oily fish, eggs, cheese, liver, butter and fortified margarine.
Vitamin E	'Safe intake' is at least 3mg for women and 3mg for men	A powerful antioxidant, which helps to protect the body cells from potentially harmful free radicals (see page 73). Also aids immunity.	Vegetable oils, seeds, nuts, avocados, sweet potatoes, green vegetables, eggs, whole grains.
Calcium	700mg	Reduces risk of osteoporosis by helping to build then maintain strong bones (and teeth). Also helps to regulate nerve and muscle function, blood clotting, the immune system, hormone secretion and blood pressure.	Milk and dairy products, pulses, bread, green vegetables, canned sardines, calcium-fortified soya milk and orange juice, dried fruit.

Iron	14.8mg for women, 8.7mg for men and women after the menopause.	Protects against iron-deficiency anaemia – the most common of all nutritional deficiencies – as it is a key component of haemoglobin in red blood cells which carries oxygen from the lungs to other body cells where it's used to produce energy.	Meat and meat products, liver, oily fish, shellfish, fortified and whole grain breakfast cereals and breads, pulses, nuts, seeds, green vegetables, dried fruit. Vegetarian should note that iron is not very well absorbed from non-meat sources – this can be boosted by a vitamin C rich food or drink at meals (see page 72).
Magnesium	270mg for women, 300mg for men	Helps give rigidity to bones and release energy from food. Needed for healthy nerve and muscle function, immunity and mood regulation.	Nuts, pulses, green vegetables, sunflower seeds, fish and seafood, dark chocolate, whole grains, bananas, dairy foods and meat.
Potassium	3,500mg	Helps regulate blood pressure, heartbeat, nerve and muscle function.	Vegetables, fruit, juices, potatoes, pulses, whole grains, nuts, seeds, fish, milk, meats.
Selenium	60mcg for women, 75mcg for men	Important part of antioxidant enzymes made in the body and plays a role in cancer prevention, reproduction, mood regulation and thyroid function. Many of us have low intake and could benefit from including good sources regularly.	Brazil nuts, other nuts, fish, seafood, meat, offal, poultry, lentils, cheese, eggs, whole grains.
Zinc	7mg for women, 9.5mg for men	Involved in the sense of taste and smell, immune function, wound healing, sperm production, foetal development, night vision, insulin production and skin health.	Oysters and seafood, meats, milk and dairy foods, pumpkin seeds, eggs, pulses, nuts, whole grains, sweetcorn.

Note: RNI (Reference Nutrient Intake) given is the UK recommended daily intake for adults.

Making the most of fruit and vegetables

- Slice fruit on to your breakfast cereal.
- Go continental and start your main meals with a salad.
- Add extra vegetables to casseroles, soups, curries and pasta sauces.
- Keep some fruit handy as a convenient, naturally packaged snack.
- Top frozen or chilled pizza with extra sliced vegetables before heating, and serve with a green salad.
- Fill around half your plate with salad or vegetables.
- Enliven crisp salads with exotic fat-free or low-calorie dressings. Balsamic vinegar with added garlic is great.
- Top stewed or canned fruit in juice with low-fat custard or fromage frais.

- Indulge in exotic tropical fresh-fruit salads – you won't need any cream.
- Enjoy the natural flavours of steamed vegetables and skip the butter.
- Measure just a teaspoon of oil for stir-fry vegetables and spice up with soya or other low-fat sauces.
- Store fresh vegetables in the fridge and steam or cook them lightly to preserve precious nutrients.
- Low-fat fromage frais makes a mayonnaise alternative for coleslaw and potato salads – why not spice up with some curry powder?
- Serve vegetable sticks with dips in packed lunches and as anytime snacks.
- Seasonal produce from markets helps with food budgets, as can the 'there when you need it' convenience of frozen and canned produce.
- Organic produce is available, but the choice is yours. There is no clear evidence that it has a nutritional advantage over standard produce.

MEAT, FISH, EGGS, PULSES AND MEAT ALTERNATIVES

Key Nutrients Protein, B vitamins, zinc, selenium, magnesium, iron, potassium, iodine. Phytochemicals in beans, lentils, nuts, seeds, tofu.

Lean meat is a very nutritious food and an important source of key nutrients such as protein, iron, zinc and B vitamins. But meat can be very fatty, especially if it is processed into sausages, burgers or pies, so choose carefully. Nutritious alternatives to red meat include poultry (watch the fatty skin), fish, eggs, pulses (peas, beans, lentils), Quorn, tofu, nuts and seeds, so there's plenty of choice in this group for vegetarians or people who eat little or no meat.

Fish is an especially good source of a number of nutrients that our diets are often short of. These include magnesium, selenium and iodine, and beneficial omega-3 fats which are provided by oily fish such as mackerel, sardines, salmon, trout, pilchards and herrings (see page 84). Pregnant women should take special note. Omega-3 fats are important for a baby's brain and eye development so if you don't eat fish, omega-3-enriched eggs, linseeds, pumpkin seeds, walnuts, soya and rapeseed oil also provide these important fats. For the sake of our hearts the Department of Health advises all of us to have fish at least twice a week and to include one portion of oily fish. Dietitians advise people who have had a heart attack or have heart disease to eat two to three portions of oily fish each week (about 200g/7oz in total).

Vegetarian alternatives such as peas, beans, lentils, tofu, nuts and seeds are good sources of beneficial fibre and phytochemicals, so try to include some of these choices too. In fact, eating nuts regularly (about 28g/1oz, two to five times a week) has been linked to a reduced risk of heart disease and heart attack.

Aim to have 2–3 portions a day. A portion could be:
- 56–84g (2–3oz) cooked meat or chicken
- 112–168g (4–6oz) cooked fish or seafood
- 2 eggs (keep to about four a week)
- 4–5 tablespoons cooked beans, lentils or tofu
- 2 tablespoons of nuts, seeds or nut butter

HOW MANY DAILY PORTIONS DO YOU CURRENTLY HAVE? _____

Make the most of meat, fish and alternatives

- Opt for trimmed, lean red meat, and chicken or fish without breadcrumbs, batter or fatty skin.
- Keep meat portions small, half fill the plate with vegetables or salad and include some potatoes, rice or pasta.
- Stir-fries and pasta sauces are delicious ways to add more vegetables and enjoy smaller meat portions.
- Use low-fat cooking methods: grill; bake or roast on a rack; microwave; poach; barbecue; chargrill or stir-fry.
- Non-stick pans and oil sprays are also useful.

- Brown meat in its own juices.
- Roast meats on an oven rack and let the fat drip into a tray.
- Have oily fish once a week – smoked, canned, or fresh.
- If you feel unsure about cooking fish, buy a simple recipe book or ask a fishmonger for advice. Barbecues, ovens and griddle pans make it easy.
- Use canned beans or tofu as a meat alternative or to make meat go further in casseroles and hearty stews.
- Enjoy eggs boiled, poached or 'fried' in a non-stick pan.
- Ensure that vegetarian meals aren't always based on cheese or pastry and do contain protein-rich foods.
- Choose lower fat versions of ready meals (ideally no more than 15–20g fat per portion).

MILK AND DAIRY FOODS

Key Nutrients Calcium, protein, vitamins B_2 and B_{12}, zinc, iodine, vitamins A and D (in non-skimmed dairy foods). Phytochemicals in soy-based milk and desserts.

Milk and dairy foods are important providers of bone-strengthening calcium, as well as protein and a wide range of other vitamins and minerals. On average they provide about 60 per cent of our calcium, so if we avoid them for some reason, it's vital to include other calcium-rich alternatives. Calcium-fortified soya milk is one, but if you really don't like it a calcium supplement (400mg – 500mg a day) is a good idea. Calcium-fortified juices and waters are also available, but they are not nutritionally similar to milk (or well-fortified soya milks) so are not dairy replacements.

People are often tempted to avoid dairy foods when slimming, but new evidence indicates that low-fat ones as part of a balanced diet may actually help us to control our weight. We also need to be especially careful to ensure a good calcium intake while slimming to protect our bones. So think twice before cutting back.

The good news is that lower fat versions, for example, skimmed and semi-skimmed milk, low-fat yoghurt and fromage frais, Edam, Brie or half-fat Cheddar are still excellent sources of calcium. These are healthy choices because they are lower in cholesterol-raising saturated fat. Aim to have 2–3 portions of dairy foods daily (teenagers need 3–4).

A portion is:
- A glass (200ml) of milk or calcium-fortified soya milk
- 35g (1¼oz) hard cheese – small-matchbox size
- 125g (4½oz) cottage cheese
- Small pot (150g) yoghurt, fromage frais, custard or rice pudding

HOW MANY DAILY PORTIONS DO YOU CURRENTLY HAVE? _____

Make the most of milk and dairy foods

- Buy semi-skimmed or skimmed milk – they have as much calcium as full-fat milk.
- If you love strong-flavoured hard cheese use small portions in cooking or in sandwiches to stretch the taste further. Grated Parmesan is a great example – 1 tablespoon adds loads of flavour for just 45 calories.
- Experiment with low-fat fromage frais as a topping, in cooking or mixed with soft or canned fruit for a snack.
- Look for low-fat or 'virtually fat free' flavoured yoghurts.
- Try low-fat soft cheeses and flavoured cottage cheese.
- Make white or cheese sauce with low-fat milk and thicken with cornflour rather than butter and flour.
- Goat's cheese, Brie, Jarslberg, Camembert, ricotta, feta, halloumi, mozzarella and Edam cheeses are all medium in fat – making them a better choice than hard cheese – but still keep to small amounts.

FOODS CONTAINING FAT AND FOODS CONTAINING SUGAR

Key Nutrients Fat and sugar, with some essential fats and minerals, and vitamins such as vitamin E in vegetable oils.

These are the foods we 'hate to love' and 'love to hate' because the fat and/or sugar they contain makes them irresistibly more-ish. Fat 'carries' flavour and adds 'mouthfeel' to food. Thanks to our hunter-gatherer ancestors, we are born with a natural liking for calorie-rich sweet and fatty foods (once upon a time we needed to store those calories when we could). This also means we have to sort of learn to like everything else – no wonder kids go for crisps and sweets if they have the choice!

Cooking oils, spreads, sugar, cake, biscuits, jams, confectionery, pastries, rich sauces, crisps and sugary drinks fall into this group. They don't need to be avoided but all that fat and sugar (and often salt) does mean that if you are serious about managing your weight they are best eaten in very small amounts. And preferably not at the expense of more nutritious foods from the other four food groups.

You will, of course, eat some foods in this group, such as oils and spreads, on most days. Choose types rich in monounsaturated or polyunsaturated fats and low in cholesterol-raising saturates (check labels) and use them very sparingly. Low, 'light', or reduced-fat versions of spreads are an ideal choice. A reasonable portion would be about three to four teaspoons each day. Keep butter for special occasions.

Rich sauces, biscuits, luxury ice cream, sweets and crisps, are best limited to small amounts, say one to two daily portions – a portion could be two biscuits, a small chocolate bar, a slice of cake, scoop of ice cream, small packet of crisps – as part of your balanced diet.

HOW MANY DAILY PORTIONS DO YOU CURRENTLY HAVE? _____

Making the most of foods containing fat or sugar

- If you are using a moist sandwich filling or a toast topping (such as baked beans) skip the butter or margarine. Pickles, chutney, tomato sauce and mustard make low-fat alternatives.
- Buy low- or reduced-fat spreads which are high in monounsaturates or polyunsaturates and low in saturates (less than 16g saturates per 100g spread) – and spread very thinly.
- Remember that olive and other unsaturated oils are as high in fat and calories as lard or butter, so use sparingly.
- Try oil-free salad dressings, make your own low-fat versions or measure oil-based dressings out with a spoon.
- Beware 'low-fat' versions of cakes, biscuits and ice creams. These often contain extra sugar so aren't much lower in calories than standard versions – check labels carefully.
- Also beware – fat in foods like pastries, processed meats, dressings, ready meals, crisps, nuts, sweets, ice cream and biscuits. Compare labels and choose those lowest in fat.
- Instead of cakes and biscuits try dried or fresh fruit, bread sticks, rice crackers, rice pudding or yogurt, a mini fruit-bun or slice of malt loaf.

ALCOHOL

Enjoying a drink can be sociable and relaxing and may even benefit our health. The famed Mediterranean style of eating, for example, includes a modest amount of wine (but is also rich in heart-healthy fruit, vegetables, fish, pasta, nuts, garlic and olive oil). However, drinking too much is not good for our health or waistlines. Good intentions tend to fly out of the window after a few drinks and too much booze could make us more apple shaped. So bear in mind current 'sensible' daily limits. These are 2–3 units for women and 3–4 units for men.

A unit is:

- Half a pint of standard beer, lager or cider
- A small glass (typically 100ml–125ml) of wine
- A pub measure (25ml) of spirits
- A 50ml glass of sherry or port

Alcohol is a toxin and above sensible limits it is a continuously increasing risk to health. Binge drinking is bad news, and sensible daily limits were set to discourage units being saved up. If you do exceed the healthy limit it's wise to have one or two alcohol-free days. This is, anyway, a good thing to do. 'Hazardous' drinking is defined as 15–35 units a week for women and 22–50 units a week for men. Above these upper limits, drinking is 'harmful'. The short-term problems include bad hangovers, moodiness, time off work, and an increased risk of injury and car accidents. In the long term, regularly drinking too much greatly increases the risk of alcohol dependency, low fertility, high blood pressure, vitamin and mineral deficiencies, cancers of the digestive tract, heart disease, liver disease, depression and osteoporosis. Eek!

HOW MANY DAILY PORTIONS DO YOU CURRENTLY HAVE? _____

Making the most of alcohol

- Quench thirst with water.
- Alternate alcoholic with non-alcoholic drinks.
- Choose low-calorie mixers and have with single measures of spirits.
- Beware 'alcopops' – they are packed with sugar.
- Keep creamy cocktails for those really special occasions.

COMPOSITE FOODS AND EATING AWAY FROM HOME

Of course, a lot of the foods we eat are not single items but composite meals or dishes that involve a number of foods from different groups.

Lasagne, sandwiches, meat and vegetable casseroles, fish pie and rice pudding are some classic examples. Then there are ready meals, takeaways, pizzas and so on.

With composite foods or meals, all you need to do is apply the same principles you would to a meal of single items. In the case of a ham and mushroom pizza, the base is from the breads and cereals group, the ham from the meat group and the cheese from the milk and dairy group. The mushrooms and tomato purée will provide some vegetables, but for a balanced meal you would need to have the pizza with a salad.

Making healthy choices from within the food groups is important. While chip-shop chips are from the bread and cereals group, they are much fattier than non-fried potatoes, so it's best not to have them too often. The same goes for things like meat pies, sandwiches dripping with mayonnaise, battered fish and creamy chicken kormas.

FATS OF LIFE

We all need some fat in our diet to stay healthy. It provides us with the fat-soluble vitamins A, D, E and K, and also with 'essential' fats that the body can't make and which must therefore be supplied by our diet. But most of us eat too much of it for our health's sake, especially cholesterol-raising saturated fat. And because fat is a very concentrated source of calories, keeping your fat intake down is one of the most effective ways to control your weight. Fat is also not very good at helping us to feel full, which makes it easy to unwittingly overeat when high-fat foods are a normal part of meals or snacks.

You may hear about 'good' and 'bad' fats. This basically means that it is not just the amount of fat that can affect health, but also the type. Remember, though, that while some fats are healthier than others they are all high in calories. Moderation is the key and healthy daily limits are 95g of fat for men and 70g for women. This equates to around 33 per cent of calories coming from fat. The limit is higher for men as, on average, they need more calories than women. If you are slimming, a fat-intake closer to 30 per cent of calories is usually recommended. So the recommended daily fat intake would be around 50g if you are keeping to about 1500 calories. (30 per cent of 1500 = 450 ÷ 9 = 50, remembering that 1g fat contains 9 calories.) Note that this is hardly a fat-free diet, so 'low fat' doesn't mean that extremes are required!

Fats are made up of building blocks called fatty acids. No food or oil has just one fatty acid, they contain a mixture of different ones. The four types you may hear about are:

- **Saturates** Eating too many can raise blood cholesterol levels, which in turn may increase the risk of heart disease. Foods high in saturates include fatty meat, lard, butter, cream, hard cheese, full-fat milk, pastries and rich ice cream. Healthy recommended daily limits are 30g for men and 20g for women.

- **Monounsaturates** In moderation, monounsaturates have beneficial effects on blood cholesterol levels, especially if used in place of saturates. Foods rich in monounsaturates make a healthy choice, and include olive oil, rapeseed oil, spreads made from these oils, peanut oil, avocados and most nuts.

- **Polyunsaturates** Some polyunsaturates are 'essential' and there are two families: omega-6 and omega-3. Both families are needed for growth, building cell membranes, brain development and to help regulate functions such as blood clotting, blood pressure and immunity. In moderation, omega-6 polyunsaturates help to lower blood cholesterol levels and omega-3 polyunsaturates help to reduce the risk of heart attacks. Omega-6s are found in sunflower, corn, safflower and soya oils and margarines; and sunflower and sesame seeds. Omega-3s are found in oily fish (the best source), liver, eggs, seafood, rapeseed oil, walnut oil, spreads made from a blend of olive and rapeseed oil, pumpkin seeds, wheatgerm, walnuts, tofu and omega-3-enriched foods. The balance between the omega-6 and omega-3 families can also influence our health. Since we get plenty of omega-6 fats in our diet – in spreads, oils and processed foods – it's best to limit these and shift the balance with foods and oils high in omega-3s.

- **Trans fats** Most trans fats are by-products of a chemical process called hydrogenation, which makes unsaturated fats firmer. Like saturates they can raise blood cholesterol levels, so are best limited. Trans fats are found in hard margarines and other foods that contain hydrogenated fats (check labels), fast food, pastries, biscuits, cakes, butter, full-fat milk and meat.

SWEET AS SUGAR?

Sugars, like starches (found in bread, pasta, rice, potatoes, cereals, etc.) are forms of carbohydrate. There are many different types: fructose is naturally found in fruit and honey; sucrose, or what we know as 'sugar', is extracted from sugar cane and beets; lactose is the sugar in milk. Glucose is the simplest form and, as well as being part of most sugars, it is the basic building block of starch. It is also the type of sugar that circulates in the blood – known as 'blood sugar' – and provides the body with energy. Most forms of sugar end with the letters 'ose', so look out for hidden forms of sugar when checking ingredient lists.

Sugar and Health

Sugar is not in itself 'bad for you', but if you eat too much your diet could be less nutritious as pure forms of sugar provide calories without any other nutrients. The main health problem directly linked to sugar is tooth decay. Bacteria in the mouth use sugars to produce tooth-damaging acid and eating sugary foods too often puts teeth at risk.

There is currently a lot of debate about the effect sugar may have on obesity, as well as insulin resistance (see page 14). Sugary foods can only make us gain weight if they cause us to eat more calories than we burn. Since sugar, especially when combined with fat, makes food taste wonderful (think chocolate, cakes, ice cream, biscuits, puddings), it's no surprise that it's easy to consume too many sugar-packed calories.

When it comes to insulin resistance, if you are not very active and also overweight frequent sugar-rich snacks may well make insulin resistance worse by keeping insulin levels pumped up and contributing to unhealthy levels of fats in the blood. But those effects won't make you gain weight, because you can only store fat if your calorie intake is higher than your needs. If you lose some weight, limit sugar and become more active, your body can use insulin more efficiently and the levels of fat, glucose and insulin in your blood will also improve.

A modest amount of sugar can be part of your balanced diet, even if you are slimming. One level teaspoon of sugar weighs 4g and contains 16 calories. Recommended limits for women are 50g (12 teaspoons) and for men 70g (17 teaspoons) of added sugar each day – which includes sugars in honey, jam, fruit drinks and processed foods as well as the sugar you add to food. These amounts are based on calorie intakes of 2000 for women and 2500 for men. If you are slimming, they would be proportionally less – for example, 38g (9½ teaspoons) for someone keeping to around 1500 calories.

We are born with a liking for sugary foods. Knowing that it's OK to have something sweet when we really fancy it can help us to feel more satisfied with our dietary changes. This means we're less likely to be thrown off course by negative thoughts like 'I've eaten that "bad" food so I may as well keep on going'! So, a little of what you fancy may well do you some good.

FIBRE – THE INS AND OUTS

We've all heard enough jokes about fibre to last us a lifetime, and it's still hard to avoid picturing a mound of raw bran when we hear the word. Fibre, a form of carbohydrate, stays largely undigested by the body, with the result that much of it literally goes 'in' and then 'out'.

The health-promoting foods in which it comes naturally prepacked (whole grains, fruit, vegetables, nuts, seeds) do a lot of good along the way. Fibre-rich foods don't just keep us regular, they also help to protect us against a wide range of short- and long-term health problems. There are two main types of fibre:

▪ **Insoluble fibre** This is found mainly in bran-based cereals, wholewheat bread and pasta, and vegetables. It acts a bit like a sponge, soaking up water in the bowel, and making the contents soft and bulky and stimulating natural bowel movements. This helps to prevent constipation and other related disorders such as diverticular disease, piles, and some cases of irritable bowel syndrome (however, some people with IBS need to limit their fibre intake). Fibre absorbs fluid, so drink at least 1.5 litres (6 – 8 glasses) of fluid each day to ensure that the fibre can do its job properly.

▪ **Soluble fibre** This is mainly found in pulses, oats, barley, rye and most fruits. It forms a gel-like gummy mixture that slows the digestion and absorption of food and its nutrients. This helps to regulate the level of glucose in our blood and control cholesterol levels. It may also regulate appetite by helping us to feel fuller for longer. Foods rich in soluble fibre tend to have a low glycaemic index (GI) (see below).

Fibre can also benefit the balance of bacteria in the bowel. Fibre and resistant starch (a type of starch that resists digestion) pass into the colon (large bowel) where they are broken down to varying extents by natural gut flora: the billions of bacteria that naturally dwell down there and help to maintain health.

THE GLYCAEMIC INDEX

The glycaemic index (GI) is an ideal example of how the healthy eating message has been 'fine-tuned' as nutrition knowledge unfolds. It is a ranking of foods from 0 to 100 that indicates how quickly a food will raise blood glucose levels. The rankings are compared to glucose, which has the GI of 100. Carbohydrate-rich foods that are digested quickly have the highest GI rankings, as they rapidly raise blood glucose levels and trigger a quick release of insulin into the bloodstream – to bring the blood glucose back down to a stable level. In contrast, carbohydrate-rich foods that are digested more slowly have a more sustained effect on raising blood glucose levels. These have low GI rankings and stimulate a lesser and more gradual insulin response. This seems to have a number of health benefits, including a stabilizing influence on blood glucose, and appetite. In other words, low-GI foods supply slow release, satisfying energy. While research is still in its infancy, diets rich in low GI foods may also help us to regulate our weight, probably because of their satisfying effects on appetite.

People with diets rich in low GI foods also tend to have a lower risk of developing problems like heart disease and type 2 diabetes. And if you look at the list (opposite) of key low-GI foods you will see that they are predominantly whole grains, vegetables and fruits – consistent cornerstones of a healthy diet.

The simple way to enjoy low-GI eating is to make a low-GI food part of a meal. This will help to lower the GI of the meal or snack overall. This doesn't mean that nutritious foods with a high GI, for example white or wholemeal bread, potatoes, rice or tropical fruits should be avoided. But when you eat them, combine them with a low GI food: baked beans on white or wholemeal toast; a glass of orange juice with Shredded Wheat; a chilli-bean filling for a baked potato; a low-fat fruit yoghurt after a wholemeal sandwich.

Foods with a Lower GI

Oats, muesli, bran-based cereals, pulses (peas, beans, lentils), sweetcorn, Basmati rice, pasta, noodles, sweet potato, cracked wheat, rye bread, heavy granary and fruit bread, pitta bread, non-tropical fruits and juices, dried fruit, low-fat yogurt and custard.

The glycaemic index of some popular foods

To determine a food's GI it must be carefully tested in a laboratory for its effect on blood glucose levels.

Food	GI	Food	GI
Glucose	100	Kidney beans, canned	52
Baked potato	85	Orange juice	50
Cornflakes	81	Baked beans	48
Wholemeal bread	71	Spaghetti, white, cooked	44
White bread	70	Orange	42
Sucrose (table sugar)	65	All Bran	42
Rye crispbread	64	Apple	38
New potatoes	62	Yogurt, low fat, fruit	32
Pineapple	59	Lentils, cooked	30
Basmati rice	58	Peanuts (but watch their	
Porridge	58	calorie and fat content)	14
Multigrain bread	55		

Source: Adapted from Foster-Powell K et al 'International table of glycaemic index' AJCN, 2002

SALT - SHAKE THE HABIT

Everybody needs a little salt, but on average we consume twice as much as the healthy limit. Cutting back can help to lower raised blood pressure – as can being a healthier weight, being more active and limiting alcohol – which in turn reduces the risk of stroke, heart disease, heart failure, and eye and kidney problems.

For most people, raised or high blood pressure (greater than 140/90mmHg) is a 'silent' disorder, yet it affects around one in three British adults. If it runs in your family, of if you have diabetes or are very overweight, have it checked regularly.

Our liking for salt is very much down to habit. No more than 7g of salt a day for men and 5g for women is recommended. Try these tips if you would like to have a healthier salt intake.

- Around three-quarters of the salt we eat comes from processed foods, so cook with fresh ingredients whenever possible.
- Look out for 'unsalted', 'no added salt' and 'salt reduced' canned and packaged foods.
- Limit or avoid added salt when cooking or at the table.
- Use herbs, spices, garlic, wine, lemon juice, vinegar and tomato purée to add natural flavours to cooking.
- Eat plenty of fruit and vegetables and include whole grains. They are excellent sources of the mineral potassium, which helps to counterbalance sodium and regulate blood pressure.
- Salt, is salt, is salt. Rock, sea or vegetable salt – they are all forms of salt.
- Salt substitutes will help you to cut back on, but not avoid, salt. Note that they aren't suitable for people with kidney disease.
- Food labels often list salt as sodium, as salt is made of sodium chloride.
- To convert sodium measures to grams of salt, multiply the sodium value by 2.5. For example, 2g sodium = 5g salt.

DRINK UP

While we can survive for weeks without food, we can only last a matter of days without fluid. This is because around two-thirds of the body is made up of it. Fluid is constantly lost when we sweat and breathe, as well as in urine and through bowel movements. This means we lose even more fluid when the weather is hot or when we are exercising (we sweat more to keep the body cool). Central heating and air conditioning can also increase our fluid needs.

Some fluid is found in food (as water), but to replace the constant losses most people need to drink at least 1.5 litres (six to eight glasses) of fluid each day. This could double in hot weather, or when you're being very active. The best way to check that you are drinking enough is to note the colour of your urine. If it is a light straw colour that's fine; if it is dark and in small quantities you need to drink more.

Water is a cheap, convenient, calorie-free way to meet our fluid needs. But we can vary it with other drinks. The best choices include sugar-free soft drinks and squashes, a glass of pure fruit juice or low-fat milk, herbal teas, or a few cups of tea or coffee. Many soft drinks and flavoured waters have added sugars so, as always, don't be fooled by labels and marketing hype – read the nutritional information. Remember pure juice is high in natural sugars too.

Some people swear by drinking eight glasses of water a day to manage their weight. If it works for you, then go for it. Certainly, drinking water before a meal may help to take the edge off your appetite – and sometimes people confuse thirst with hunger, and eat when what their body really wants is water. The main thing is to drink enough fluid, and make sure you aren't undoing good efforts by drinking lots of sugar, and fat, in the process.

What about supplements?

Most of us can meet our nutritional needs with a full and varied diet. However, busy lives can mean that we don't always eat as well as we would like to.

Some women don't get enough minerals such as iron (especially if they have heavy periods), selenium and magnesium in their diet. Men tend to do better, but again may run short on some minerals (though rarely iron). In these cases, an 'insurance policy' of a one-a-day multivitamin and mineral supplement with amounts of vitamins and minerals close to the recommended daily allowances (RDAs) can be a safe addition to your diet. The same is true when you are slimming. You may also want to consider a supplement if your diet is restricted in some way. For example, if you are allergic to dairy products, and find it difficult to eat enough alternative calcium sources, it is wise to take a daily calcium supplement (400–500mg). If you are vegan you need to ensure that you get vitamin B_{12}, calcium and iodine from fortified foods or supplements each day, since animal-derived foods are the best sources of these nutrients.

Official health advice is that when planning to have a baby, and for the first 12 weeks of pregnancy, women should take 400 micrograms of folic acid daily to help protect against neural tube defects such as spina bifida. Pregnant and breastfeeding women are also advised to take a 10 microgram vitamin D supplement, especially if their skin's exposure to sunlight is limited (the action of sunlight on the skin forms vitamin D in the body). If you are pregnant, or planning pregnancy, please remember to check the suitability of any supplements – especially those containing vitamin A – with your doctor or midwife before taking them.

While supplements can help to prevent nutritional deficiencies, they can't replace all the health-regulating and disease-combating effects of food. It seems that it's not just specific vitamins or minerals that protect our health – real food brims with a wide range of natural antioxidants and nutrients that work together to provide us with optimal nutrition for long-term health and well-being.

KEY FOOD TIPS FOR HEALTHY WEIGHT CONTROL

There's no doubt that a few key points stand out about weight control. Making healthy food choices certainly helps us to cope better with the toxic environment, but it also helps our health and well-being in many other ways. So what's good for our weight, is also good for nourishing body, mind and soul.

Despite ongoing research into diet and weight control, we still can't say that there is one optimal composition for a diet. There are advocates for diets ranging from low carbohydrate, high fat to the opposite extremes of very low fat and high carbohydrate. What is most likely, is that different approaches may suit different people – and even these may vary between periods of actively losing weight and maintaining a stable weight. But research also suggests that, for long-term weight-control success, behaviour change rather than diet composition alone is what makes the difference. So once more we are back to the importance of individualized, sustainable and achievable lifestyle changes. There is more about this in Step Four.

Meanwhile, studies point towards the dietary factors that best help to satisfy the taste buds and regulate appetite, blood glucose, insulin and energy levels, and metabolism. Together, these factors make it easier to make and maintain dietary changes. If your diet is drastically different, don't worry. You can use the information in the book to change for the better – and make the most of food.

- Enjoy regular meals, starting with breakfast. Watch portion sizes.
- Eat at least five portions of fruit and vegetables daily.
- Make starchy carbohydrate-rich foods, especially whole-grain types, part of meals.
- Make low-GI foods part of meals and planned snacks.
- Have moderate portions of low fat protein-rich foods at meals.
- Include two to three portions of low-fat dairy foods daily.
- Limit foods with a high energy density – such as ones high in fat and refined carbohydrate.

ENERGY DENSITY OF FOODS

On average, our bodies like to consume a fairly regular weight of food. Nutrition scientists suggest that around 2kg (4¼lb) each day is most likely to keep us satisfied, and habit nibbling at bay. It therefore makes sense, if we are trying to control the amount of calories we consume, to get most of this weight from those foods with a low 'energy density'.

This means ones with a low concentration of calories per portion – in other words, more bulk per calorie.

This is achievable with a balanced selection of foods in line with the 'Balance of Good Health' – as opposed to a diet of burger meals, when our calorie needs would be met after eating only 700g (1½lb) of food – leaving us feeling empty and wanting more!

Vegetables, fruit, low-fat milks and yoghurts, whole grains, pulses (peas, beans and lentils), lean meat, chicken and fish are the best foods, as are dishes made using them, such as vegetable soups, meat, fish or bean and vegetable casseroles, pasta with tomato-based sauces and fruit-based desserts.

See what you can get for 150 calories

- 17g (1⅕ tablespoons) of oil
- 20g (4 level teaspoons) of butter or margarine
- 40g (8 level teaspoons) of low-fat spread
- 230g (4 medium boiled or 1 large baked) potato
- 54g (half a regular serving) of French fries
- 28g (one small packet) of crisps
- 40g pretzels
- 30g (4 small squares) of milk chocolate
- 625g (7½ portions) of steamed broccoli
- 320g (3 whole) apples
- 37g (1⅓oz) of hard cheese such as Cheddar
- 75g (2½oz) of fresh goats' cheese
- 40g (5 tablespoons) of sugar-frosted-flakes cereal
- 47g (6 tablespoons) of bran flakes
- 400g (2 medium bowls) of vegetable soup

step three

part two

EATING DIFFERENTLY

Now that your knowledge about healthy eating has been refreshed, and you've had the chance to see how your diet currently measures up, the next step is to make some changes to the amounts you eat. This doesn't necessarily mean eating less of everything. In fact, for many people it means eating more of some foods. This probably makes eating differently sound easier than it is. As you will well know if you have tried changing your eating habits before, it can be difficult. But it can be done. And no doubt you have your own important reasons to want to make the change.

This section has two parts. The first focuses on setting goals that will help you make practical, and realistic, changes to your eating habits. It is about how small changes add up to make a big difference. The second provides a more structured eating plan, and gives clear guidance on portion sizes, balance and overall calorie control. There is, however, a common theme linking the two, which is also directly relevant to the physical activity part of your lifestyle change. And that's the fundamental skills of cognitive behavioural therapy (CBT, see page 53). They will help you to deal with 'why' you are finding it hard to achieve and maintain a healthier weight. This is different to so many diet plans that simply focus on what you have to do to get to some goal weight, almost regardless of anything else! You will learn the necessary skills, knowledge and motivation en route to your goals and, when you find your healthier weight, use them to stay there.

Weight-Loss Basics

Now for a quick recap on how we lose weight. Love them or hate them, calories do count. But that doesn't mean you have to count them constantly. It does help, however, to have a feel for both the calorie content of foods and your calorie needs. This is especially helpful when you are buying ready prepared and labelled foods. Or when you are snacking on high fat foods like cheese or crisps!

Basically, if we take in fewer calories than we burn we tap into our fat stores and gradually lose weight. If we cut around 500 calories each day, we can lose a pound a week (a pound of fat contains 3500 calories, and 7 x 500 = 3500). This means something has to change foodwise. But how it is done is up to you. It's a matter of keeping your food diary (see page 53) as carefully as you possibly can, identifying what changes are most likely to make a difference and setting SMART goals for change (see page 56). Sometimes a few food swaps are enough to make a difference (see below). Or some small but regular changes, like using less oil in cooking (1 tablespoon of oil has 100 calories) and less spread on bread every day, might be enough to make a difference by themselves. You decide!

Eat differently – and swap it

The small changes you make can really add up. Achieving food changes could be as simple as getting used to making a few healthy swaps over the day – for example, switch to semi-skimmed milk and reduced calorie dressings, swap a chocolate bar for fruit or choose 'light' rather than full-fat yoghurts. Here are some examples. Also write down any swaps you think of that suit your eating habits better – and test them out. You can check the calorie content on the pack, or use a good calorie-counting guide.

☐ Swap chips for boiled or baked potatoes (no butter) – Save 300 calories.

☐ Swap a BLT for a 'healthy choice' BLT – Save 270 calories.

- ☐ Swap a chocolate bar for a banana – Save 150 calories.
- ☐ Swap a pint of full-cream milk for semi-skimmed – Save 120 calories.
- ☐ Swap a glass of lemonade for diet lemonade – Save 60 calories.
- ☐ Swap a large ready meal of vegetarian lasagne for a calorie-controlled portion – Save 450 calories.
- ☐ Swap normal dressing on a salad for oil-free – Save 90 calories.
- ☐ Swap a 200g pot of flavoured yoghurt for 'light' yoghurt – Save 100 calories.
- ☐ Swap standard coleslaw for reduced-calorie coleslaw – Save 240 calories per small pot.
- ☐ Swap a restaurant pepperoni pizza for ham and mushroom pizza – Save 165 calories.
- ☐ Swap a takeaway sweet and sour chicken with egg fried rice for stir-fried beef with green pepper and black bean sauce and steamed rice – Save 610 calories.
- ☐ Swap a takeaway chicken korma with half a naan and pilau rice for chicken dupiaza with chappati and plain rice – Save 605 calories.
- ☐ Swap a large burger with small fries and regular cola with cheeseburger, small fries and diet cola – Save 550 calories.
- ☐ Swap a double vodka and energy drink for a double vodka and low-calorie tonic – Save 115 calories.
- ☐ Swap a 175ml glass of sweet wine for a 175ml glass of red or dry white wine – Save 50 calories.

Making Changes

You may find it helpful to change either the amounts you eat of certain foods or the types of food – or a bit of both. Or it could be your eating style that causes you problems. Below is a list of the sorts of changes many people find helpful. Have a look through them and tick the ones that might help you. Some may not be relevant – for example, you don't eat red meat or drink alcohol, or you are already following some of the guidelines – so just ignore those. Then use your food diary, and what you know about your own habits to write down any other changes that would help to address why you find it difficult to manage your weight.

Remember to be realistic. These changes will become your key weight-control goals. Test them out one or two at a time, to see if you find any unsuspected barriers and if they do indeed really help you to eat differently. People often find that it helps to make a note when they achieve a goal. Use the SMART guidelines to keep your goals achievable and relevant and so build your confidence in your ability to change. If the going gets tough, refer back to your reasons for wanting to make these changes and lose weight. And use the skills still to come in Step Four, to help you stay on top of slimming saboteurs.

Possible Changes

Eating Differently – Types, Amounts and Cooking Methods

When 'portions' are mentioned, look back to the 'What is a healthy diet?' section on page 64 for guidance.

1   Use low-fat cooking methods – grill, stir-fry, bake, microwave, barbecue, stew – rather than frying or cooking with a lot of added fat.
2   When you do use a small amount of oil in cooking, measure it with a teaspoon (one per person) or use an oil spray.
3   Trim the fat from meat before cooking and remove the skin from poultry (most of the fat lurks there).
4   Buy lean mince and lower fat versions of any sausages or burgers.
5   Keep red meat portions modest – no more than 112g (4oz) in a day.
6   Have fish at least twice a week.
7   Make one of these servings an oily fish, e.g. mackerel, sardines, trout, salmon, pilchards. If you use canned versions, avoid those in oil.
8   If you are vegetarian, have meat alternatives each day, e.g. peas, beans, lentils, eggs, tofu, Quorn, or some nuts or seeds.
9   When buying ready meals, choose those with no more than 450 calories and 20g fat per portion – serve with extra vegetables or salad.

10 Have at least six to eight glasses/cups/mugs of fluid each day. Look for soft drinks with no added sugar. This includes water, but not alcohol!

11 If you have sugar in tea or coffee – cut it out (gradually if you prefer).

12 Have at least two alcohol-free days each week.

13 Keep within healthy alcohol limits (see page 81) – on most days of the week at least!

14 Have two to three servings of low-fat dairy foods daily.

15 Limit your cheese intake to 112g (4oz) per week.

16 If you use full-fat milk, switch to skimmed or semi-skimmed milk.

17 Have low-fat and no-added-sugar yoghurt, mousse or fromage frais (often described as 'diet' or 'light') rather than full-fat versions.

18 Use a low- or reduced-fat spread rather than full-fat butter or margarine – and still use very sparingly.

19 Think twice before using cream. Could you use low-fat plain or fruit yoghurt instead?

20 Buy oils rich in unsaturated fats, e.g. olive oil, rapeseed oil, soya oil, peanut oil – and use sparingly (see point 2).

21 If buying sandwiches, look for types with no more than 350–400 calories per pack.

22 Limit high-fat and/or sugar snacks, e.g. packet of crisps, small chocolate bar, piece of cake, two biscuits, to one portion a day.

23 Serve yourself three or more portions of vegetables or salad daily (half-fill your plate at your main meals).

24 Use an oil-free salad dressing or just a little (about 2 teaspoons) standard dressing.

25 Try out a vegetable or fruit that's new to your shopping list, each week.

26 Have at least two to three portions of fruit each day.

27 Keep to one small glass of pure fruit juice each day – this can count as one portion of fruit.

28 When buying canned fruit, choose types in juice rather than syrup.

29 Have some vegetable or fruit nibbles such as carrots, celery, red peppers, melon, strawberries in the fridge at home, and at work. Sugar-free jelly,

a glass of tomato juice or a mug of vegetable soup can also be helpful.

30 Make some starchy carbohydrate, e.g. rice, pasta, potatoes, cereal, bread, crispbread, noodles, part of your meal.

31 If you eat out more than once a week (this includes lunches as well as dinners), use the eating out guide to make wise choices (see page 122).

32 Use a healthy eating recipe book for new ideas and inspiration. Write down your own goals for changing the types and amounts of food that you eat.

Eating Behaviour

Step Four has more detailed information about many of these goals.

1 Keep up your careful food diary each day.

2 Have three regular and planned meals (see page 102).

3 If you like to have snacks, plan two or three into your eating plan.

4 Keep your meals to a similar size each day.

5 Have breakfast every day – or at least within two hours of getting up.

6 Do not miss meals, even if you have overeaten at another meal that day.

7 Sit down when you eat.

8 Sit down to eat at the same place at home (and at work if possible) and only eat when sitting there – not on the run, in the car, in bed or in the bath! Make this your 'eating only' place too, and aim not to use it for any other activity.

9 Eat without any other distractions, e.g. turn the TV off and don't read or listen to a radio programme. Instead, pay attention to your meal – the taste, texture, enjoyment. People who do this feel more satisfied and so control how much they eat more easily.

10 If you normally serve food on large dinner plates, use a smaller one to help control portion sizes and keep the serving looking generous.

11 Serve your portions, then clear away and store or freeze any leftovers before you sit down to eat, rather than putting the leftovers on the table or within easy reach while you are eating.

12 Eat slowly and chew your food well. Put your knife and fork down in between eating if that helps.

13 Take at least 15 to 20 minutes to eat your meal.

14 With your evening meal, always try to leave a little on the plate – to overcome the 'I must clean my plate' mentality.

15 Leave the table feeling just comfortable, rather than full. It takes a good 15 minutes for your brain to get the message that you've had enough.

16 Clean your teeth after breakfast and your evening meal.

17 Don't go shopping when you are hungry.

18 Plan meals for the week ahead. Use a food shopping list.

19 When shopping, take time to check and compare the calorie and fat content of foods. If you wear reading glasses, take them too!

20 If you know·you will be busy in the coming week buy quickly assembled or 'ready' meals and/or cook a large dish, e.g. a casserole, pasta sauce, divide it into meal-size portions and freeze.

21 Appreciate that cravings can be a normal response to the fact that food is everywhere, and is seductively advertized. Help yourself by keeping it behind cupboard doors and being choosy about the food and cookery items you read and watch on TV. Don't have 'problem' foods in the house – at least until you feel more in control of your eating.

22 If you overeat, try not to tell yourself off or give up. Instead, plan how you might deal with a similar situation differently next time.

23 Prepare a list of distracting activities to take your mind off food e.g. do some gardening, paint your nails, go for a walk, call a friend, work in the shed, take a bath, do some housework. Or it may suit you better to acknowledge and 'surf' the craving (see Step Four).

24 Recognize that we all eat in response to different 'triggers' – boredom, learned habit, negative thoughts, hunger, a social event, stress or unpleasant feelings. Seek help with learning how to cope differently with these situations rather than feeding them (see Step Four).

25 Beware of aiming for perfect eating. This is unrealistic, unnecessary and not much fun! Instead aim for flexible restraint (see page 147).

   Now make a note of your own goals for changing things about your eating behaviour

Why Eat Regular Meals?

Eating regular meals is something we're always advised to do, but the reason why it helps so much is rarely explained. Regular meals and planned snacks help you to spread your food intake over the day. Regular eating is also perhaps the most important step towards breaking free from the often destructive cycle of overeating and strict dieting (see page 68). If we frequently follow rigid diets, skip meals due to lack of time, or eat for comfort we override our natural hunger and feeding signals. This makes it difficult for our bodies to recognize when they need nourishment, and how much. The end result can be bingeing, high-fat snacking or nibbling all night long after a day of eating little.

However, a regular meal pattern on a day-to-day basis enables you to get back in tune with natural feelings of hunger and fullness. This is because it helps to keep your blood sugar levels stable (this is also good for your mood and for heart health) and to think less about food between meals – because you don't feel too hungry and know that another meal is coming soon. A regular meal pattern also seems to help your to body to learn when it's time for your next meal; and lets you recognize when you have had enough to eat more readily, and so stop eating.

PERSONAL WEIGHT-CONTROL GUIDE

If you like more structure and information about portion sizes than is given in the goal-setting approach, this personal weight-control guide is for you. Or you may already have made use of many of the goals, improved your diet and lost some weight, but would like to lose some more. Your personal meal planner will help you to eat around 600 calories less than your current calorie needs – the number of calories that would keep your current weight stable. If your planner is combined with some extra daily activity you can lose up to 0.9kg (2lb) a week. This is a steady and well-balanced loss, and is an approach that is frequently used in large clinical studies into obesity. It is also widely used by dietitians and doctors working with people who want to control their weight.

The planner should be used in combination with the other skills described in this book – including the goals for changing eating behaviour (see page 95) – to enable you to make lifestyle changes that you can keep up. This is vital if you want to not just lose, but also to keep off, the excess weight that is currently affecting your health.

Note: If you are under 18, breastfeeding, are not overweight, have a medical problem or take medication, please check with your doctor before following any weight-loss plan, including this one. Weight loss is not recommended during pregnancy.

The planner is not a rigid diet, and requires portion and calorie 'awareness' rather than calorie counting (I've also done most of that for you). It allows you to plan and choose meals and so develop your own effective weight-loss plan. Please note that all values are as accurate as is practical and necessary, but they are not 'exact'.

There will be times when you wander away from the plan. We all like to have a curry or a good meal out now and then, or a bit of party. You can be flexible and maybe 'bank' some extras for planned indulgences. At other times life, habit or emotions might simply take over. If so, don't see this as a failure. It isn't. It's natural. And worrying about it could make you want to keep on eating and give up (if this is a regular problem, see Step Four for advice).

If you have got this far you have no doubt made up your mind that you want to lose weight, and are focused on just that. See each meal as an opportunity towards achieving what you want. Remember all the reasons why you want to make changes, picture yourself at your new realistic weight, and stay on track for your pleasurable journey. Keep your food diary up too – it will be a vital part of your success.

Calculating the Right Calorie Level for Your Weight-Loss Needs

You can approximate your basic calorie needs with scientifically tested calculations that make use of your current weight, age, sex and activity level. How to carry out these calculations is explained below. Once you have your calorie level for weight loss, you can use the charts to find servings from different food groups, which will be the basis of your meal planner. See the example and the food exchange system below the calorie and servings guide.

First decide on your physical activity level according to the descriptions below. This decides your Activity Factor. If you aren't sure, it's best to go for a lower level.

- Inactive = Activity Factor of 1.3 (Spend most of your day and evening sitting)
- Light = Activity Factor of 1.4 (Some day-to-day activity, e.g. for example, moving around at work, housework, cooking, general tasks, some walking.)
- Moderate = Activity Factor of 1.5 (Spend much of your time on your feet each day rather than sitting, or do regular exercise, e.g. jogging, a gym workout, sports or dance training, at least three or four times a week.)

Now calculate your resting metabolic rate – the number of calories you would burn in a day if you were lying still and not doing anything (see page 37). **Note**: 2.2lb = 1kg; 1 stone = 6.4kg.

Age Range (Years)	Men RMR (calories/day)	Women RMR (calories /day)
18–30	15.3 x weight (kg) + 679	14.7 x weight (kg) + 496
30–60	11.6 x weight (kg) + 879	8.7 x weight (kg) + 829
60 plus	13.5 x weight (kg) + 487	10.5 x weight (kg) + 596

Calories burned each day = RMR x Activity Factor

Calorie level for steady weight loss = RMR x Activity Factor – 600

- An example is a 37-year-old lightly active woman (she has an office-based job and walks to work and back but does no other regular exercise) who weighs 79kg (12stone 7lb).
- Her RMR is 8.7 x 79 (= 687) + 829 = 1516
- As she is lightly active, multiply by her Activity Factor of 1.4 to calculate the approximate number of calories she currently needs to keep her weight stable.
- 1516 x 1.4 = 2122 (round down to 2100).
- Now, to lose weight, she needs to eat less, so subtract 600 calories (2100 – 600) = 1500 calories, which will be her calorie target for steady weight loss.

Use Calorie Ranges or Do Your Own Thing

If these calculations sound a bit complicated, why not choose a calorie level and see how it goes? Most women will lose a pound or two a week if they have 1400–1600 calories a day, and most men will lose steadily on 1800–2000 calories a day. Remember, the heavier and more active you are, the higher your calorie needs. So if you are very overweight, go for a higher calorie level rather than being tempted by a lower one. You will still lose weight, and because your meal plans will be more satisfying, they will be easier to keep to. See page 113 for some quick and easy calorie-counted meal ideas.

You can use the structure of the food exchange system to plan balanced and portion-controlled daily eating patterns. Or, if you prefer to do your own thing, use your calculated calorie level as a guide for developing your own eating plan, or to help you judge how pre-packed sandwiches or meals, or recipes (with calorie information, that you follow) fit into your overall day.

Using Food Exchanges and the Meal Planner

Use your calorie level to plan your food choices and meals with the exchange lists below. If your calculated calorie level for steady weight loss is higher than any of the values shown, you may find that the goal-setting approach is a better place to start (see pages 95–102). Or ask your doctor to refer you to a local dietitian for individualized advice.

FOOD EXCHANGE GUIDANCE

Calorie levels and numbers of servings from each food group

	1200	1300	1400	1500	1600	1700	1800	1900	2000	2100	2200	2300	2400
Starchy	*5	5	5	6	6	6	7	7	8	8	9	9	9
Fruit	2	2	3	3	3	3	3	3	3	3	3	4	4
Vegetables	4	4	4	4	4	4	4	4	4	4	5	5	5
Meat	*4	5	5	6	6	7	7	8	8	8	8	9	9
Milk	2	2	2	2	2	2½	2½	2½	3	3	3	3	3
Fat	3	3	3	3	4	4	4	4	4	5	5	5	6
Extras	50	100	100	100	150	150	150	150	150	200	200	200	250

* Or swap to make 4 starchy and 5 meat servings if you prefer.

YOUR MEAL PLANNER

Fill in the gaps according to your requirements as listed above.

Recommended servings for your personal eating planner (to provide a daily total of ___calories)

____ Starchy (breads, potatoes and cereals)

____ Fruit

____ Vegetables

____ Meat (including vegetarian alternatives and fish)

____ Milk (and dairy foods)

____ Fat (spreads, oils and dressings)

____ Extras (calories for planned snacks)

FOOD GROUP EXCHANGES

Use the following lists to add variety and interest when you plan your regular meals and snacks. The portion sizes are there to guide you especially while you are getting used to the meal plan; you don't need to measure things constantly. But in the toxic environment, where 'big portion sizes' are rife, getting it right can make a big difference. And don't forget to choose lower GI foods from the exchange lists to make part of your meals whenever possible (see page 88).

Starchy – Breads, Potatoes, Cereals	1 serving
Breakfast cereal	3 tablespoons or 1 Shredded Wheat/Weetabix
Porridge oats, muesli	2 tablespoons (to make into porridge)
Bread, any variety	1 medium slice (around 36g)
Roll, bagel, English muffin	Half
Large tortilla wrap, pitta bread	Half
Crumpet, Scotch pancake, mini pitta bread	1
Pure rye crispbreads	3
Rice cakes	2
Pasta, egg noodles, couscous	3 rounded tablespoons/half a cup, cooked (28g/1oz uncooked)
Rice, barley	2 rounded tablespoons, boiled (28g/1oz uncooked)
Boiled potato	1 medium or 2 egg-sized
Baked jacket potato	Half a medium potato
Oven chips	6 chips
Thin pizza base	Quarter of a medium pizza base
Kidney or other beans	3 heaped tablespoons
Sweetcorn	1 corn on the cob
Thick vegetable soup	Medium bowl

| 'Cook in' sauce, non-creamy | 1 portion |
| Plain popcorn (popped with no fat/sugar) | 3 cups |

Protein Foods   1 serving

These are cooked weights for meat, fish and beans (uncooked weights for meat, poultry and fish will be 25 per cent bigger).

Lean beef, pork, lamb, chicken, turkey	1 thin slice or 28g/1oz
Ham – no fat	42g/1½oz
Chicken casserole	56g/2oz
Bolognese sauce or chilli	56g/2oz
White fish, seafood or Quorn	56g/2oz
Oily fish e.g. mackerel, trout	28g/1oz – aim to have once a week
Fish finger, low-fat sausage	1
Bacon	1 lean rasher
Egg	1
Beans, lentils, baked beans, tofu	2 tablespoons
Lentil or bean soup	Half a medium bowl
Nuts, seeds, nut butters	1 level tablespoon (14g/½oz)
Hummus, reduced fat	1 rounded tablespoon

Vegetables   1 serving

Aim to half-fill your plate with salad or vegetables and make vegetables or fruit part of every meal or snack. Have more if you like – these servings are to encourage you to eat enough, rather than limit the amount!

Any vegetable except potato, beans and corn	2–3 heaped tablespoons
Salad	Dessert-bowl-sized side salad
Tomato	1 medium tomato or 4 cherry tomatoes
Tomato puree	Portion for pasta

Fruit	1 serving
Medium fruit, e.g. apple, orange, pear	1 fruit
Banana	1 small
Berries	1 cupful
Grapes	Small bunch (approx 12)
Small fruit, e.g. satsumas, plums	2 fruit
Large fruit, e.g. melon	Large slice
Canned/stewed fruit	3 tablespoons
Fruit juice	125ml glass
Dried apricots	3

Milk and Dairy Foods	1 serving
Skimmed milk	285ml (½ pint)
Semi-skimmed milk or soya milk (with calcium)	200ml (⅓ pint))
Low-fat natural or 'light' yoghurt, fromage frais or soya dessert	Small pot (around 90–100 calories)
Hard cheese, Brie, Edam	28g (1oz)
Low-fat soft cheese	56g (2oz)
Cottage cheese	2 heaped tablespoons/small pot

Fats and Oils	1 serving
Margarine, butter, spread	1 level teaspoon
Vegetable oil	1 level teaspoon
Low-fat spread	2 level teaspoons
Low-fat salad cream	1 tablespoon
Single cream	1 tablespoon
Mayonnaise	1 teaspoon
French/Italian dressing	2 teaspoons
Oil-free dressing	2 tablespoons

Snacks/Extras – these are suggestions only. Add more to the lists if you like.
Around 50 calories
1 fruit serving
1 'slim' soup or 1 mug of low-fat vegetable soup
1 portion low-fat 'cook in' sauce/1 tablespoon curry paste
Crudités with 2 tablespoons salsa
Small pot of 'diet' fruit yoghurt
1 level scoop of low-fat ice cream or sorbet
1 plain biscuit or meringue nest
1 low-calorie hot chocolate drink
1 pub measure of spirits (25ml) plus low calorie mixer
85ml glass of dry wine – plain, or as a spritzer with some ice and soda

Around 100 calories
Any 2 fruit servings
200g/7oz pot 'light' yoghurt or one other dairy serving
1 slice of bread with thin low-fat spread and yeast extract
2 crispbreads with scraping of peanut butter or low-fat soft cheese
1 slice of garlic bread
1 mini fruit bun or cereal bar
1 fun-sized chocolate bar or chocolate biscuit or 2 plain biscuits
Small bag of savoury snacks (around 100 calories)
150ml glass of wine or half-pint of beer, cider or lager or
    1 (25ml) liqueur

Around 150 calories
1 wholemeal salad roll
1 fruit bun or scone
150g pot low-fat rice pudding or custard
150-calorie dairy dessert or yoghurt
1 small packet of crisps
1 small chocolate bar (28g/1oz)

1 medium cereal bar (28g/1oz)
Bottle of beer or 2 small (100ml) glasses of wine

Around 200 calories
1 extra bread and 1 extra dairy serving
2 crackers plus 28g/1oz cheese
Small bowl of breakfast cereal with semi-skimmed milk
1 fruit serving plus cereal bar or packet of crisps
2 fun-sized chocolate bars
200-calorie snack, cake or dairy dessert
Pint of beer, stout or lager
Two (150ml) glasses of wine

Drinks
Have at least six to eight drinks over the day. Choose from: water,
mineral water, sugar-free squashes and soft drinks, herbal tea, tea or
coffee with milk from the exchange lists.

Miscellaneous
It's a good idea to enhance the natural flavours of your cooking with
calorie-free or very low calorie seasonings and sauces. Try adding
dried and fresh herbs, spices, garlic, fresh chilli, lemon or lime juice,
flavoured vinegars (especially balsamic), tomato purée, a good-
flavoured stock, a splash of red or white wine, sherry, soya sauce, hot
pepper sauce, teryaki sauce, capers, a few olives and mustards.

Supplements
A one-a-day multivitamin and mineral supplement is advised for meal
plans with less than 1900 calories.

Putting Meals Together Using Exchanges

Hummus and Salad Wrap – per wrap

1 tortilla wrap – 2 starchy servings
2 tablespoons of low-fat hummus – 2 meat/alternative servings
Salad – lettuce, sliced peppers, spring onion, tomatoes – 1 vegetable serving

Chicken Stir Fry – for the whole meal (serves 4)

Chicken –500g (1lb 2oz)
Sliced mixed vegetables, e.g. onions, peppers, mushrooms, baby corn, snow peas
1 tablespoon of oil plus spices – to taste, e.g. garlic, ginger, chilli or soya sauce

Serve your portion with 4 heaped tablespoons of boiled rice. The meal will provide:
2 starchy servings
2–3 vegetable servings
3 meat/alternative servings
1 fat serving

Ham and Mushroom Pizza with salad – half a medium (350g/12oz) thin-based pizza

2 starchy servings (from the pizza base)
2 vegetable servings (top with extra peppers and tomatoes)
2 meat/alternative servings (from the ham)
1 milk and dairy serving (from the cheese)

▪ Pre-packed sandwiches/snack meals – choose types that provide around 300–500 calories, depending on your total calorie intake.
▪ Ready meals – in place of a main meal. Choose meals with around 400–500 calories and serve with extra vegetables or salad.

Your Exchange Check List

To keep track of your meal planning, it can help to keep a checklist of your food exchanges. You could make it part of your food diary. Simply write down what you eat and tick off the exchanges you have at each meal and snack, as shown in the example below.

Time	Food/Drink	Exchanges for 1500 calories						
		Starchy	Protein	Fruit	Veg	Dairy	Fats	Snacks
8 a.m.	Orange juice			1				
	6 tbsp branflakes with milk	2				½		
	Milk for hot drinks over day					½		
10 a.m.	Apple			1				
	White tea							
1 p.m.	Pitta bread	2						
	2 tbsp hummus (reduced fat)		2					
	Side salad, dressing				1		1	
	Light yogurt					1		
	Fizzy water							
3 p.m.	White tea							
	1 ginger biscuit							50-ish
7 p.m.	Chicken & veg stir-fry		4		3		2	
	Rice – 4 tbsp	2						
	Canned peaches			1				
	1 scoop low fat ice cream							50-ish
9 p.m.	White coffee							
Total for the Day		6	6	3	4	2	3	100
Target		6	6	3	4	2	3	100

QUICK AND EASY MEAL IDEAS

Breakfasts (around 350 calories)

- Small glass of fruit juice. 1 cup of preferred cereal with semi-skimmed milk. 3 dried apricots.
- Toasted bagel spread with low-fat cream cheese. Small glass of fruit juice.
- Small glass of fruit juice. 2 slices of wholemeal toast with low-fat spread and jam or honey.

- Smoothie – blend 1 cup soya or semi-skimmed milk with 2 tablespoons natural yogurt, 1 large banana or 3 canned peach halves.
  Add 2 teaspoons wheatgerm (optional) and honey to taste.
- Small glass of fruit juice. Boiled egg. 2 slices of bread and low-fat spread with yeast extract as soldiers.
- Small glass of fruit juice. 4 tablespoons baked beans on toasted muffin.
- 1 small pot plain yoghurt, with 3 dried apricots and 5 almonds (chopped). 1 mini fruit bun.
- Small glass of fruit juice. Wholemeal roll with peanut butter or cheese spread. Apple.
- 2 small sausages (grilled) or 2 slices lean-back bacon served with grilled tomato, 2 slices wholemeal bread and brown or tomato sauce.
- Small glass of fruit juice. Bowl of hot-oat cereal, with semi-skimmed milk, banana and 1 level tablespoon raisins.

Lunches (around 400 calories)

- Canned or smoked salmon in 2 slices granary bread. 2 pieces of fruit.
- 2 slices wholemeal bread filled with with 1 tablespoon peanut butter mixed with low-fat soft cheese and cucumber. Bunch of grapes.
- Pasta and feta salad made with 3 tablespoons (56g/2oz) cooked penne, cubed feta cheese, 4 olives (chopped), fresh basil, cherry tomatoes and cucumber and 1 tablespoon of fat-free dressing. 1 portion of fruit.
- Baked jacket potato filled with tuna in brine ($\frac{1}{2}$ a small tin) and 2 tablespoons low-calorie coleslaw. 1 satsuma.
- Mini pizzas made with either a split white crusty roll or medium pitta bread spread with a mixture of garlic and tomato purée, topped with half-fat Cheddar cheese and grilled. 1 portion of fruit.
- Any type of pre-packed sandwich or 'snack meal' (around 300–350 calories). 1 portion of fruit.
- 2 slices cold roast beef served with lettuce, tomato, cucumber salad and oil-free dressing. Chunk of French bread. 1 banana.

- Ciabatta bread filled with a small tub (112g/4oz) of low-fat cottage cheese (plain or flavoured), mixed-leaf salad and 1 tablespoon oil-free dressing.
- Plain hamburger or cheeseburger. 'Regular-size' orange juice.

Dinners (around 450 calories)

- Grilled fillet steak (150g/5oz uncooked weight) served with carrots, sprouts, 3 medium potatoes (boiled) and 2 tablespoons gravy. 3 tablespoons stewed or canned apples with 1 tablespoon fromage frais.
- Portion of cod in parsley sauce served with broccoli, carrots and 10 oven chips. 1 portion of fruit.
- Smoked mackerel (90g/3½oz) served with tomatoes, green beans and 4–5 new potatoes.
- Warm chicken salad made with 125g/4½oz of chicken stir-fried in 1 teaspoon olive oil and herbs/spices of choice. Serve with mixed-leaf salad (with 1 tablespoon oil-free dressing) and 1 medium pitta bread. Canned fruit in juice with 1 tablespoon fromage frais.
- Garlic and mushroom thin-base pizza topped with extra sliced peppers, mushrooms and tomatoes, served with salad and oil-free dressing.
- 2 grilled vegeburgers served with a medium jacket potato, 1 tablespoon low-fat fromage frais, 2 tablespoons baked beans and 1 grilled tomato. Small bunch of grapes.
- Mushroom omelette (2-egg) cooked in 2 teaspoons olive oil served with tomato salad and 1 wholemeal roll (no spread). Individual mousse.
- Pork kebabs (125g/4½oz uncooked meat) skewered with cherry tomatoes, green pepper and mushrooms, marinated in sweet and sour sauce, grilled and served with 4 tablespoons Basmati rice and green salad. Fruit salad.
- Stir-fried chicken or Quorn (125g/4½oz uncooked weight) cooked with 1 teaspoon olive oil, garlic, ginger and vegetables served with 1 cup of boiled noodles. 200g pot of 'light' fruit yogurt.

step three

part three

SMART SHOPPING

When you buy fresh foods you know what you are getting. But today we also have a vast range of processed foods to choose from. And unless we know what we are buying, it's all too easy for these foods to push us into the clutches of the toxic environment. The good news is that many of them are fine in your healthy diet – remember, all foods are 'legal' – but some label-reading know-how will help you to make the best choices.

When comparing labels consider how the food might fit into your overall diet. Ingredients are always listed in descending order of weight, so the first on the list is there in the greatest quantity, and the last in the least. Some foods may be high in sugar, fat or calories, but if you only eat them very occasionally – for example, cheesecake as a birthday treat – they can fit into the balance of your diet. The Daily Guideline Amounts are a useful guide (see page 68). Eating foods such as ready meals, dressings, milk or canned fruit regularly, or in larger amounts, affect your diet more, so it's worth looking for types that are lower in fat, sugar and calories.

Beware big packs of food, unless you have a big family to feed. They may save a bit of money, but if they make it difficult for you to control how much you eat any cost benefit is lost. It helps to avoid aisles crammed with foods you are trying to eat less of, and to take a planned shopping list with you. Also, try not to shop when you are hungry, tired, depressed or stressed.

A good nutrition label lists nutrients per 100g of food and also nutrients per typical portion. It may also show how many portions there are in the pack, so make sure you aren't eating all of a pack that is actually meant to serve two. Also make sure that what you tend to serve yourself isn't bigger than the typical portion size. Always checking your portion sizes (see page 126) will stop you getting more than you bargained for.

Guideline Daily Amounts

Guideline daily amounts have been approved by the Department of Health to help us see how a particular food fits in to a healthy diet. They are average values, for people with an 'average' weight and activity level, who are aiming to keep their weight stable. In the case of fibre, the figure is a recommended minimum intake. If you are reducing your calorie intake, your guideline intakes will be proportionally less (see the 1500 calorie column below) as an example.

When shopping, you can compare a food's nutrient content to the following average values. For example, if a ready meal contains 40g fat and 3g salt it is very high in both of these (over half a woman's daily limit), so not a healthy choice. If you do decide to eat it, you will then need to balance it with low-fat and salt choices over the day.

Each day	Men	Women	
Calories (kcal)	2500	2000	1500
Fat (g)	95	70	50
of which saturates (g)	30	20	16
Salt/sodium (g)	7/2.5	5/2.0	3.8/1.5
Added sugar (g)	70	50	38
Fibre (g)	20	16	12

Nutrition Claims

Many foods carry nutrition claims as well as nutrition information. There is currently no legislation about such claims, simply official guidelines. This is what some of the more common ones *should* mean.

- Low fat – no more than 3g fat per 100g food.
- Reduced fat, sugar or sodium – 25 per cent less fat/sugar/sodium than in a standard version of the food.
- High fibre – at least 6g fibre per 100g food.
- % fat free – these claims are discouraged. If something is '90% fat free' it is still ten per cent fat, so is not a low-fat food.

Lower Fat Alternatives

Here are some foods where hidden fat abounds, and some sleeker alternatives. Some people like to look for foods with no more than 5g fat per 100g. This is OK, but can be a bit restrictive if applied to all foods, especially if you only eat a very small amount of the food or eat it very occasionally. Less than 10g fat per 100g is perhaps more realistic, with no more than 20g of fat for a whole meal, for example in a ready meal.

Half a pint (285ml) milk for tea and coffee. Swap full cream – 187 calories, 11g fat with semi-skimmed – 130 calories, 4.5g fat
- Save: 57 calories, 6.5g fat

Breakfast

Swap a plain toasted bagel with butter and jam – 482 calories, 20g fat – with 2 medium slices of wholemeal toast, with thin low-fat spread and reduced sugar jam and a small glass of juice – 300 calories, 8g fat
- Save: 182 calories, 12g fat

Lunch

Swap a standard bought BLT – 540 calories, 26g fat – with a 'healthy choice' BLT (with lean bacon and low-fat mayo) – 270 calories, 14g fat
- Save: 270 calories, 12g fat
Swap a 40g packet of crisps – 211 calories, 13.5g fat – with a 28g

packet of 'light/low fat' crisps – 135 calories, 6.5g fat
- Save: 76 calories, 7g fat

Swap a can of standard cola – 130 calories – with a can of diet cola – 2 calories
- Save: 128 calories

Snack
Swap a chocolate bar – 250 calories, 14g fat – with 1 banana and 1 apple – 150 calories, 1g fat
- Save: 130 calories, 13g fat

Evening meal
Swap pasta with carbonara sauce and a mixed salad and liberal dressing – 890 calories, 52g fat – with pasta with a non-creamy chicken arrabiata sauce, 1 tablespoon grated Parmesan and mixed salad with low-fat dressing – 660 calories, 20g fat
- Save: 230 calories, 32g fat

Swap a large glass (250ml) of medium white wine – 185 calories – with a 175ml glass of dry white or red wine – 115 calories
- Save: 70 calories

Swap 3 cream crackers with cream cheese – 199 calories, 13g fat – with 3 water biscuits with reduced-fat cream cheese and a slice of melon – 140 calories, 6g fat
- Save: 59 calories, 7g fat

Totals
Standard meal plan: 3075 calories, 122g fat
Modified meal plan: 1900 calories, 60g fat
SAVE: 1175 calories and 62g fat – and eat just as much, if not more!

ADAPTING RECIPES AND FAMILY MEALS

If you have a family cooking separate meals for yourself is not practical or helpful. Simply adapting family favourites means you don't just have the opportunity to enjoy them, you also lead by example and help the whole family to healthy eating habits.*

* Under-fives often have small appetites. They should have varied diets, but not low-fat diets, to ensure they meet their nutritional needs.

1   Plan meals ahead for the whole week, if possible. Make a shopping list based on your plan.

2   Cooking vegetables:
- Retain flavour and vitamins by steaming or microwaving vegetables – then serve as soon as they are cooked.
- Mash potatoes with milk and skip the butter. Add extra flavour with sliced onion, cabbage, mustard, fresh herbs or olives, or other mashed vegetables like carrots or swede.
- Top baked potatoes with natural or 0% fat Greek yoghurt, fromage frais or flavoured cottage cheese rather than butter or margarine.
- Try 'dry roasting' potatoes. Boil them for 10 minutes, drain, and shake the saucepan just once. Then remove the potatoes, place on a baking tray (spray with a little oil spray if you like) and 'roast' as usual.

3   Making sauces.
- Make a gravy using gravy powder and water, rather than meat juices.
- Use low-fat milk as a basis for a white sauce, and thicken with cornflour rather than butter and flour (make a paste by mixing 1 tablespoon of cornflour with 2 tablespoons of skimmed milk. Heat 600ml (1 pint) milk until just boiling then stir in the cornflour paste, bring back to boil, stirring continuously, and cook until thickened). For cheese sauce, use a small amount of strong cheese such as Parmesan or blue cheese.

- Tomato or vegetable-based sauces, rather than creamy ones, are ideal for pasta.
- If buying sauces, look for brands with less than 5g fat per 100g.

Adapting recipes

Shepherd's Pie
- Cook minced beef (or try turkey, soya or Quorn mince) in a non-stick saucepan (with a little oil spray if needed) over a low heat.
- Stir continuously to stop sticking. Drain off any fat.
- Add finely chopped onions and any other favourite flavourings e.g. herbs, tomatoes, spicy sauce.
- Try some canned kidney beans too.
- Top with mashed potato, made with low-fat milk, then bake.

Tuna or Salmon Pie
- Use fish canned in water or brine (drain well).
- Make a white sauce as described above – if you like, flavour with parsley or mustard.
- Add some peas, canned beans and/or corn for filling fibre.
- Top with mashed potato, made with low-fat milk.

Lasagne
- Cook the mince as for the Shepherd's Pie or swap the mince for canned tuna, Quorn or soya mince (and cook with canned tomatoes, chopped vegetables and herbs)
- Make the cheese sauce as described above.

'Creamy' Pasta Sauce
- Mix 1 level tablespoon grated Parmesan into 2 level tablespoons low-fat fromage frais, then toss through hot cooked pasta shapes.

Honey 'Cream' Topping

* Blend together a 250g pot of ricotta cheese, 1 tablespoon honey and 1 teaspoon vanilla essence. Use as a topping for fruit salad or to fill a meringue nests.

Grill-Up

* If you like to linger over a Sunday cooked breakfast, then slash calories and fat by grilling a sausage, lean back-bacon slice and tomato, poaching an egg and serving with beans, a slice of whole-grain toast and a glass of orange juice. *Bon appetit!*

EATING OUT

We all like to treat ourselves from time to time, which is just wonderful. But these days eating out has become a regular part of life. The trend worries obesity experts who feel that it's a key contributing factor to the UK's ever-growing obesity problem. This may be because when we eat out we have much less control over how the meal is prepared and how big the portions are. To help us feel that we are getting good value, they are usually larger than the ones we would normally serve. Combine this with the fact that food eaten out is generally higher in fat, and we can end up taking in far more calories than if we had eaten at home. We also get used to eating bigger meals.

American studies show that people who eat out a lot often have higher intakes of calories, fats and salt. So, to manage your weight, you need to make healthier choices from the menu. There will be times when a meal out really is a treat and you enjoy eating what you want (and now that you are making conscious choices about what you really want to eat, this may not necessarily mean big portions of everything high in fat!). Other times, it's just a meal in a toxic environment, and you will use your skills to survive it.

CHINESE

Chinese food offers plenty of scope for ordering a nutritional nightmare. The nation's favourite, sweet and sour pork, is no exception. Some dishes ooze fat, while most are high in salt. But you can make reasonable choices. Beware terms like 'battered', 'deep fried' and 'crispy'; instead opt for stir-fried fish, chicken, beef or vegetable dishes. Resist the egg or special fried rice and go for plain boiled. Watch the more-ish 'seaweed' and prawn crackers. Share portions to make them go further (see page 127) for the calorie and fat counts of popular dishes). Beware 'all you can eat' buffets, too.

INDIAN

Chicken tikka masala has been described as Britain's new national dish. But with 19g of saturated fat – thanks to its cream and ghee (clarifed butter) content – it's hardly the most healthy. So, steer clear of creamy kormas, pasandas and masalas, and limit fatty bhajis, plain poppadoms, pickles and naan. Beware the biryani, too. And watch out for oil floating on curry surfaces – leave that in the dish not on your lips! Better choices include tandoori and tikka dishes, vegetable, chicken and prawn Madras and jalfrezi, balti or dupiaza dishes with boiled rice or chapattis (see page 128) for the calorie and fat counts of popular dishes).

THAI

Thai food can be an excellent choice as long as it doesn't come drenched in coconut milk and coconut cream. These add calories and saturated fat, but little in terms of vitamins and minerals. Beware deep-fried starters, too. Clear soups, seafood salads and stir-fried dishes served with steamed or sticky rice (made with a special rice grain) are the best options – which means there's actually plenty to choose from. Be warned that 'steamed' fish may mean steamed in oil and fat, so check before you order.

ITALIAN

Creamy sauces, mozzarella 'salads', garlic bread and 'fritto' dishes are Italian foes for healthy eaters. But there are plenty of lower fat soups, salads and pasta and fish dishes to choose from, to accompany a glass of robust red. Choose simple seafood, minestrone or lean ham for starters, and opt for fish, pasta, chicken or meat without batter or creamy sauces – instead, look for the following sauces: Napoletana (tomato); vongole (clams); primavera (vegetables); *provençale* (tomato, mushroom and wine), puttanesca (tomato, olives and vegetables), prosciutto (ham and mushroom); pizzaiola (tomato and olives) and bolognese (meat) – and use the grated Parmesan cheese sparingly.

BURGERS, PIZZAS AND FISH AND CHIPS

Better choices

- Plain hamburger, cheeseburger or grilled chicken burger with orange juice or a diet drink. Share some fries with a friend. Remember size matters when it comes to burgers, so beware big and large ones. Ask if mayonnaise can be left out or swapped for a lower fat barbecue or tomato sauce.
- Thin-based pizza topped with ham, seafood or vegetables. Add extra chilli and garlic rather than fatty pepperoni or extra cheese. Choose carefully from the salad bar – many 'salads' (i.e. coleslaw) are fat-laden.
- Grilled or barbecued chicken with bread roll or potato and salad
- Falafel sandwich or shish kebab – as distinct from a doner kebab
- Ask for grilled fish when you go to a fish-and-chip shop and, if it isn't

available leave most of the batter and enjoy the moist fish inside. Ask for a small portion of chips and share. Don't forget the mushy peas.

TEX-MEX

It's all the 'bits' that go with Tex-Mex food that mount up so easily, not to mention the American-style portion sizes. Sour cream, tortilla chips, cheese, deep-fried tortillas – even nutritious guacamole – just pile on the fat and calories. Fajitas (watch the bits!), grilled fish, salads, chillis and rice (plain if available) or a soft tortilla wrap make better choices.

SANDWICHES

With the exception of foccacia and some speciality breads, most breads are naturally low in fat and packed with healthy energy from carbohydrates. Wholemeal and whole-grain varieties add extra fibre and minerals, and the amount of bread in a sandwich or roll provides two servings.

For fillings choose a lean high-protein base such as roast meat, ham, chicken, tuna, fresh or smoked salmon, prawn, egg, soft cheese, hummus or a bean-based spread. If possible, choose a filling that also includes salad or chargrilled vegetables, or include some salad or fruit as well as the sandwich. And look for moist alternatives to margarine or mayonnaise, such as mustard, pickles and fromage frais. If buying pre-packed sandwiches, go for those with 300–400 calories per pack.

TOP TIPS for Eating Away from Home

1   Have light, regular meals during the day so that you're not ravenous when you reach the café or restaurant. However, it can help to 'bank' some servings/calories for the extras you'll have.
2   If you eat out regularly go to cafés and restaurants that you know have choices that suit you. Decide what you will have before you go.

3 Shun butter on bread and garlic bread or foccacia.
4 Show some American style and say how you would like a dish cooked or served. Ask for any sauces 'on the side', so you can add them as you wish.
5 Skip high-fat pastry, deep-fried and battered foods, mayonnaise, oily dressings, butter, cream and cheese sauces.
6 Look for dishes described as 'grilled', 'chargrilled', 'poached', 'stir-fried', 'steamed', 'cooked in its own juice' or with *pomodoro* or wine sauce.
7 Half-fill your plate with vegetables or salad.
8 Go for fruit-based desserts or sorbets.
9 Watch alcohol. Quench your thirst with water; alternate alcoholic with non-alcoholic drinks, try wine spritzers and choose low-calorie mixers.

TOP TIPS for Portion Control

- Studies suggest that, on average, we can underestimate how much we eat by 25 per cent. And a lot of this could be down to bigger portion sizes in eating establishments and in supermarkets.
- Learn to 'get your eye in' as to what a healthy portion size is. Measure foods occasionally at home, and have a good look at them on plates or bowls. For example, measure a cup of pasta or 4 heaped tablespoons of rice and put it on a plate. Note how much space it takes up. Use this knowledge when you eat out.
- If you are served a bigger portion than you want, decide how much you are going to eat at the start of the meal. And don't feel you have to 'clean your plate!'
- Avoid restaurants that serve 'all you can eat' buffets – the variety will make you eat more, as will the 'need' to get value for your money.

Stop, Think and Plan Ahead

- If your work place doesn't have a cafeteria with healthy choices or there are no suitable food shops nearby, plan ahead and bring food with you to work. This is especially important if you do shift work, tend to work long hours, or are going somewhere after work, for example, to a class, the cinema or the gym.

- Keep fruit at work, in the car, or in your bag or briefcase each day, so that it's to hand when you need a snack.

Calorie and Fat Counts for Popular Chinese and Indian Dishes

Calorie counts are based on typical portions from takeaways and in restaurants. This information is a guide only, since restaurants serve different portion sizes and use different amounts of added fat.

Chinese

Prawn crackers – 385 calories, 15g fat for a bowl (approximately 15 calories each)

Seaweed (per plate) – 720 calories, 67g fat

Sesame prawn toasts – around 70 calories, 7.5g per small square

Meat spring roll (55g) – 125 calories, 9g fat

Whole portion of spare ribs – 875 calories, 64g fat (so just have one!)

Chicken and sweet corn soup – 100 calories, 1g fat

Crispy duck, made into 4 pancakes – 650 calories, 36g fat

Sweet and sour chicken – 585 calories, 30g fat

Sweet and sour pork (battered) – 715 calories, 42g fat

Chicken chow mein – 515 calories, 25g fat

Stir-fry beef with green peppers and black bean sauce – 375 calories, 20g fat

Stir-fry vegetables – 185 calories, 14g fat

Szechuan prawns with vegetables – 310 calories, 17g fat

Chicken chop suey – 390 calories, 21g fat

Chicken with cashew nuts – 530 calories, 35g fat

Egg-fried rice – 550 calories, 15g fat (73 calories, 2g fat per tablespoon)

Steamed rice – 410 calories, 4g fat (40 calories, 0.5g fat per tablespoon)

Indian

Poppadom: plain, fried – 65 calories, 5g fat
Poppadom: spiced, grilled – 27 calories, 0.2g fat
Onion bhaji (2 medium) – 350 calories, 27g fat
Meat samosa (2 medium) – 335 calories, 24g fat
Chicken korma – 660 calories, 51g fat
Chicken tikka – 240 calories, 9g fat
Chicken tikka masala – 550 calories, 40g fat
Lamb rogan josh – 505 calories, 35g fat
Vegetable balti – 290 calories, 28g fat
Chicken biryani – 985 calories, 44g fat
Chicken dhansak – 505 calories, 30g fat
Chicken jalfrezi or dupiaza – 415 calories, 27g fat
Prawn Madras – 400 calories, 29g fat
Pilau rice: per portion and (per tablespoon) – 290 (60) calories, 5g (1.1g) fat
Boiled rice: per portion and (per tablespoon) – 245 (55) calories, 2.4g (0.5g) fat
Chappati – 110 calories, 0.5g fat (made without fat)
Naan – 540 calories, 20g fat – but size varies a lot

Average Calorie and Alcohol Counts

	Calories	Units
½ pint standard stout, bitter, lager	85	1
½ pint extra strong lager	168	2.5
Bottle of premium lager	100–150	1.5–2
½ pint standard dry cider	100	1
Bottle of 'alcopop'	150–250	1.5
125ml glass of champagne	95	1.5
125ml glass of red or dry white wine	85	1.5
175ml glass of red or dry white wine	120	2

125ml glass of sweet white wine	120	1.5
25ml spirits	50	1
25ml liqueur	80	1
50ml dry sherry	60	1
50ml port	70	1

COPING WITH SOCIAL SITUATIONS

Your social life doesn't have to stop when you start slimming. But some situations put the most resolute of us to the test. Learning skills to help you deal with different social situations is vital to the sustainable lifestyle changes that will help you to lose weight and keep it off.

Situation

'I find it hard to say "No" when people offer me food I don't feel like eating – I don't want to upset them.'

Positive response

Saying 'No thank you' is something you need to practise and feel comfortable with. Do it at home, by yourself first. It can be hard when you feel you are upsetting others, but it will get easier. If you know you are going to a friend's house for dinner, let her know in advance that you are slimming so may not eat everything. She wants to see *you*, not watch you eat! It's also easy to end up blaming others. 'She made me eat, what choice did I have?' But, of course, you do have a choice. It can help if you change the way you talk to yourself. Rather than thinking 'I must' or 'I should say no', try thinking 'I really want to say no, so I will.'

Situation

'What's the point in trying to slim? Whenever I go out I just have to eat what's put in front of me – then I feel bad and keep on eating.'

Positive response

Ask yourself: 'Is this true – why must I have this food?' 'What is the worst thing that will happen if I don't eat it?' Or, 'I could eat it if I really wanted to, and it would probably be very nice, but do I truly feel like it.' And reassure yourself with: 'Saying no will be hard at first, then the discomfort will pass as I have made the conscious choice not to eat it'. Try it out and see. This way you will start to realize that there are alternatives to your belief that you simply must eat certain foods.

Situation

'Party nibbles are my big downfall – and the more I drink, the more I nibble!'

Positive response

Not arriving hungry at a party can help to stop you scoffing the nuts and nibbles, so can standing away from buffet tables. Alternate alcoholic drinks with water to keep 'alcohol' munchies – and a hangover – at bay. Remember you are losing weight because you want to, and that not going overboard is a positive thing – not something to feel deprived about. If party mode does take over, then enjoy – and get back on track next day (once you've made it out of bed!).

step four

getting your head straight about food and weight

CHANGING YOUR MIND

If you are serious about controlling your weight, make sure you read all this section. Unless your 'head is straight' about food and weight, long-term success will be elusive. The other skills in this book will also be much less useful to you.

So what do I really mean by 'getting your head straight'? It's hard to put it into exact words, but you will know when it happens. Even though achieving it can be a slow journey for many, for some it can be like turning on a light switch. You just 'get it'. It makes sense. Your motivations become clear and powerful. Your self-esteem and self-efficacy (belief in your abilities) grow. You realize that meal plans, workouts and slimming groups might help, but that they aren't in themselves going to do it for you. You accept responsibility for what you eat and how active you are, and feel positive and empowered to make the changes you want to make. The pieces of the jigsaw start to come together.

This doesn't mean that getting your head straight becomes easy, but it becomes a more logical process that you can control. You make choices, knowing and accepting the consequences. You know you will have lapses. You use your toolbox of skills (most of the time) to stay on track and eat healthily, to be active and to take care of yourself – because you are worth it. And because it allows you to achieve your realistic goals – and reach, and stay at a weight that is healthy for you.

There is no single formula for getting your head straight. We all eat – and overeat – for different reasons. We view our bodies and our abilities in different ways. We also think and talk to ourselves differently. If you identify your unhelpful thoughts and attitudes, you can change the way you view, and respond to problems. In other words, if you want to change your weight you must first change your mind.

What is Your Relationship with Food – and Yourself – Like?

Read through the questions below and answer 'Yes' or 'No' to them

- Do you often eat to cheer yourself up?
- Do you use food to avoid confronting problems?
- Do you regularly crave certain foods?
- Does going on a diet make you feel deprived?
- Do you find yourself eating when you have time on your hands?
- Are you always trying out new diets – or thinking about doing so?
- Do you talk negatively to yourself and rarely notice your achievements?
- Do you usually eat without making a conscious choice about what you eat?
- Do you often have periods of uncontrolled bingeing?
- Do you rarely take time to really taste what you eat?
- Are you constantly dissatisfied with your body?
- Do you often get up in the night and head for the fridge?
- Do you find overeating has benefits for you?
- Does overeating make you just want to keep on eating?
- Do you eat without thinking about how physically hungry you are?
- Do you start a diet hoping it will be the one that makes you slim?

If you answered 'Yes' to more than a few, your relationship with food, and how you feel about yourself, is likely to thwart the lifestyle changes required for achieving, and maintaining your healthier weight. This section will help you to develop the skills to stop these issues sabotaging your progress. If you answered 'No' to most of them, or feel that your head is pretty 'straight', read through this section anyway, so that you know what's in it in case you find that some of the issues get in your way at a later stage.

Are You On the Right TAC for Weight Control?

You have got this far because you have decided that you really want to lose weight. Now you are taking the action that will get results. Believe it or not, our thoughts govern our every action – and their consequences. That includes what, when and why we eat, and our attitude. For example, does losing weight make you feel negative because it makes you think of deprivation; or positive because you think eating better and being more active is enjoyable, makes you feel good and enables you to achieve your much-desired goals?

The TAC system is a simple way to look at this flow of events.

T = the Trigger or situation before the event
A = our Action or response as a result of that trigger
C = the Consequence or outcome of that action or response

Going back to the example above, if the trigger is the decision to lose weight, and your thoughts go straight to deprivation, the action or response is to feel negative and the consequence is short-lived success. Alternatively, if your thoughts go to the pleasure and benefits of lifestyle changes, the action or response is to feel positive, and the consequence is to change eating and activity habits.

Or if you set a rigid rule to avoid biscuits and crisps you are more likely to feel frustrated (and overeat) than if you set a goal to choose healthy snacks. The positive approach doesn't necessarily just happen by luck or the right kind of thinking. It is more likely to be the result of going through the steps outlined in this book – deciding if you are ready to lose weight, setting realistic goals, equipping yourself with the right skills – and truly believing you can do it.

Throughout the rest of this Step, there is guidance and skill-building to help you stay on the right TAC, overcome your slimming

How we think affects how we feel

How we think about things affects how we feel about them. In turn, this feeling affects how we act or behave, and so directly influences what we do.

A man wants to learn to scuba dive, but finds the sensation of breathing under water difficult. 'I just can't get the hang of this. I am always useless at things and everyone is probably laughing at me. I may as well give up now.'
A second man wants to learn to scuba dive, but finds breathing under water difficult. 'I found it tricky today, but it is only the first time I have breathed under water, and it is bound to seem odd. The instructor said it is normal to find it a bit daunting to start with. I will see how I feel after trying it a few more times.'

How do you think each man feels as a result of his thoughts?
Which man do you think is most likely to achieve his goal?

As well as changing our thoughts and attitudes, we can also make practical changes to our environment to get us on the right TAC. Here's another example.

Jo comes home after a long day at work. She is fed up and tired. She wants a treat to revive her, so she heads for the chocolate biscuits on the kitchen counter. She eats three, quickly, without really tasting them. She now feels guilty – that she has no willpower, has blown her diet – so keeps on eating until the pack has gone.

The 'Triggers' were – coming home tired and fed up, and seeing the biscuits.
The 'Action' was – eating the biscuits rapidly and not savouring them.
The 'Consequence' was – feeling guilty, that she'd blown it, and so eating more.

Jo could have pre planned an alternative snack (if she knew she was likely to be hungry) or other ways to unwind when she got home tired and fed up (her food diary would have highlighted this as a 'problem area'). She could also have avoided keeping chocolate biscuits or similar binge foods in the house. If she had a craving for chocolate biscuits, she could have acknowledged and accepted this – but resisted it to help reprogramme the association between coming home tired and scoffing biscuits (see page 138).

Or she could change the 'action' by consciously choosing (and therefore being mindful of the consequences) to take one biscuit, make a cup of tea, put the remaining biscuits away and then sit down, out of sight of the kitchen, to really taste and savour the biscuit (aware that she can have another biscuit another time if she wants one). She would feel pleased with herself, rather than eating most of the pack, feeling a failure and abandoning her weight-loss plan.

saboteurs, and strengthen your belief in your ability to control what you eat – and your weight.

Are You Still Keeping Your Food Diary?

As highlighted by Jo's story, keeping a diary of what, where and when you eat can help you to identify and examine certain triggers, situations or feelings that make you more likely to stray from your eating plan. A diary also gives you time to stop, think and make a conscious choice (which involves thinking about the consequences of your action) about what you put in your mouth – rather than feeling as if the food is controlling you. Food diaries (see page 53) are fundamental to getting the most from this book and the skills it has to offer. And research shows that people who keep them (known as 'self-monitoring') are the ones who are most successful at losing weight.

Head Hunger versus Stomach Hunger

When I ask people what prompts them to eat, hunger usually comes down near the bottom of their list of reasons. Some of them struggle to remember or appreciate what true hunger feels like. The many reasons why we eat have already been discussed. And, typically, it isn't because we are physically hungry. One of the luxuries of our food-filled environment.

Whether it's at a meal, or at any other time of the day or night, eating when they aren't physically hungry can be a big factor in the trouble so many people have in controlling their weight. There is no perfection to aim for, though. It's fine to do some eating when you aren't hungry, but if this goes too far it's easy to overeat and gain weight (or stay overweight). One way to describe eating when you aren't hungry is 'head hunger'. The desire to eat, or overeat, is driven by triggers such as situations, thoughts and feelings – and these, rather than a physical survival-linked 'stomach-rumbling' hunger that drives us to eat, influence how we act.

How much 'head hunger' eating do you think you do? Keep a record to find out. Do this when you are still assessing your usual eating habits rather than actively changing them. Once you start to eat differently, you can use awareness of your 'head hunger' eating to help you to achieve your goals.

A useful way to learn more about your head hunger versus your stomach hunger is to assess and rank your level of hunger on a scale of 0 to 5 (see below) before you eat. Then think about and write down how 'satisfied' you feel after eating your choice of food. This can be on two levels – is your 'stomach hunger' satisfied (1, 2 or even close to a 3 on the hunger scale); and do you feel happy with your food choice, is it what you really wanted, did it hit the right spot? When you can eat for true hunger, and choose just what you feel like eating, you gain a much more positive and conscious control over what you eat.

Hunger before eating

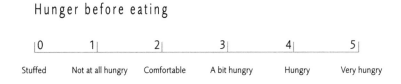

0	1		2		3		4		5	
Stuffed	Not at all hungry		Comfortable		A bit hungry		Hungry		Very hungry	

You can add extra columns to your food diary, for example:

Date *Wednesday 5 August*					
Time	Food and Drink	Where/who with	Comments	Hunger	Satisfaction?
1 p.m.	Beans on 2 slices toast with some chilli sauce	At home, alone	Fancy a hot lunch	4	Yes, hot and tasty
2.30 p.m.	Slab of chocolate cake	At home, alone	Just need something sweet	1	Feel stuffed and bad. A low-calorie hot chocolate would have done.

Consciously Choosing What You Want to Eat

If you can learn to consciously choose what you want to eat you are set to control your weight for life. This skill is like your personal 'brake'. It helps you to stop, think and act before the chips hit your hips. It helps you manage 'head hunger'. It stops you feeling deprived. It helps you to regularly remind yourself why you are making changes to your eating habits, and this keeps motivation high. But it doesn't just happen. Like all skills you have to practise it, and some people will find they have to practise more than others. Sometimes it will work well for you, at other times it won't – but overall it will help. Basically, ask yourself if you really want to eat something. This becomes the prompt for you to make a conscious choice, weighing up the pros and cons and feeling free to eat the food or reject it. In the words of a well-known weight-control motivator, 'Ask yourself if you like it enough to wear it!' Making conscious choices goes hand-in-hand with a goal-setting approach and also with more structured meal plans.

Here's an example:

Paul is having a regular business lunch at one of his favourite restaurants. He loves steak Béarnaise and fries, then *crème caramel*. But after his last medical check-up his doctor advised him to lose some of his waist for his heart's sake. He has thought a lot about changing his lifestyle. But he can't avoid business lunches. Faced with the menu, his automatic response is the steak. But then he stops and thinks. How hungry is he? How will he feel after he eats it? What would be a better and still tasty choice? After all, he comes here quite a bit so he can order the steak another time. He opts for a spicy chicken fillet with new potatoes and vegetables. He really enjoys the spicy flavour, and feels comfortably satisfied rather than stuffed and guilty. Having a dessert would just ruin the nice taste he has in his mouth and make him feel too full, so he decides against that. He is spurred on to make more changes as he now knows he can enjoy other things.

If you often feel deprived you probably aren't really making conscious choices. The same goes if you are doing a lot of 'head hunger' eating. Or maybe you are still just getting used to controlling your weight. It is hard work, having to stop and think about whether you really want to eat a meal or the food you are about to put in your mouth, thinking about the consequences of doing just that – will you feel satisfied? – and then deciding whether to eat the food, choose something else or eat nothing at all! And alongside that you have the toxic environment to deal with – the lack of healthy food choices when eating away from home, the impulse buys in service stations, the takeaways, the stress-relieving snacks. It can take time to get to grips with all this, but it can be done.

Once you've made your conscious choice, you will be ready to eat slowly and taste and savour your food. Getting the maximum enjoyment and awareness from what you eat makes the food more satisfying, with the result that you are likely to end up eating less than you might have otherwise.

Triggers for Overeating or 'Head Hunger' Eating

Overeating or eating when you aren't hungry, doesn't just 'happen', even though it might feel like it. It is the end result of a chain of events – events that have a number of triggers (see page 140). Use the TAC system to help you make the right choices, for example, next time you have the urge to eat, first stop and think:

- Ask yourself when you last ate.
- Ask where your hunger is coming from – your stomach or your head.
- If you ate a meal recently (within the last three to four hours) or don't feel 'stomach hunger', question what else might be prompting you to eat.
- Ask yourself: 'Why do I want to eat?'; 'What am I seeing or feeling?'; 'Why do I feel that way?'
- If you aren't sure why you feel that way, ask yourself 'Whatever it is that I am worried or anxious about, will eating actually change it?' 'Is there something I could do instead?'
- If you still aren't sure, think about the consequences of your action. Imagine you have just had a binge, and how it makes you feel – will it be worth feeling like that? Now imagine how you would feel if you broke away from eating this time – will it be a better feeling?
- If you do decide to eat something, make sure it's a food you really feel like. If it isn't available, would it be better to eat nothing?
- This questioning approach allows you time to identify triggers, choose whether or not you want to eat and, if you do want to eat, to choose a food that is exactly right.

Eating Triggers

Tick the eating triggers that affect how you eat and add any that aren't on the list. This will highlight your 'problem' areas.

1 External (environmental). For example:

- Watching others eat or TV cookery programmes
- The smell of food
- Walking past a cake shop
- Food advertisements and recipes
- Drinking alcohol
- Buffet meals
- Preparing food
- Eating on the run so you eat what you can get and don't savour it
- Being somewhere you associate with eating e.g. visiting your parents
- Having time on your hands
- Eating very rapidly so you can't taste the food or recognize fullness
- Skipping a meal so you get so hungry you end up overeating
- Confusing hunger with thirst
- Bad premenstrual symptoms
- Eating to please someone else
- Not having healthy foods to hand-grabbing whatever there is
- Shopping when hungry

2 Internal (linked to thoughts or feelings). For example:

- Feeling lonely or bored
- After an argument
- Feeling deprived
- Feeling stressed, anxious or tired
- Feeling fat
- Feeling frustrated with the time it can take to truly change habits

- Feeling that you deserve a reward
- Feeling low about a smaller than expected weight loss
- Feeling guilty or 'bad' about food you've just eaten
- 'Programmed' to clear your plate
- Want food to cheer you up
- Feeling angry
- Feeling that you've already blown it so you may as well keep on eating

Emotions and Eating

Successful slimmers confront their problems; they don't feed them. If you think your main triggers for overeating are emotions that affect your mood, try to identify the emotions so that you can work to find more useful ways to respond to them. Sometimes this can be difficult. It can help to talk to close friends or family members, who you know can support you best.

Relaxation exercises, walking or doing something else that you really enjoy (see page 143), can also help. As can trying to address any triggers in practical ways. For example, if you eat when you are worried about something you are trying to put off, prepare a plan of action to get it sorted. If you eat because you get lonely, or have too much time on your hands, find ways to structure your time more and to interact with people, for example, by going to evening classes or doing voluntary work. Remember, too, that it's OK to feel sad, or lonely, or angry, and you don't need to smother these feelings with anything, including food. If stress is a problem for you, read more about how to cope manage it on page 186.

If you are concerned that you may be depressed, feel that it is difficult to deal with your emotions by yourself and/or you binge a lot (see page 154), it's important that you talk to your doctor or seek help from a professional counsellor or self-help group.

'I Just Couldn't Resist It' – Coping with Cravings

Cravings may seem to 'just happen', but they're actually a normal and learned response to a certain feeling or situation – in other words, a trigger. They come on so quickly you just don't realize it. It's a bit like Pavlov's famous dogs. He rang a bell every time he fed them, and after while, whenever they heard the bell ring, they were 'conditioned' to salivate in anticipation of food.

Here are some examples of learned response cravings. If, as a child, you never went on long car journeys without travel sweets you probably automatically buy sweets for a car journey now. If your parents didn't allow you to leave the table until you had cleared your plate, you probably can't do it now. If you always see eating out as a treat, you feel you need to order the most indulgent dishes and eat as much as you can. Or if you regularly ate leftovers from the children's plates after they'd gone to school, you may get the urge to eat in response to being alone in the house.

The fact that cravings are learned means that steps can be taken to reprogramme your response to the situations or feelings that trigger them – and remember how to TAC (see page 133). It certainly helps to identify when cravings strike. Your food diary will no doubt highlight such times. The skill is to stop and think when you get that strong urge to eat. One of four things could then happen:

1   You recognize or confront the craving. The main thing is to talk to it in some way, acknowledging that it is a learned response and that you are the one in control.

2   You 'surf' the craving and if need be use a distraction method to take you away from the food situation (see opposite).

3   You eat all the food you crave (being prepared to accept the consequences, such as feeling bloated, or disappointed that you strayed from your plan).

4   You eat some of the craved food and, half-way through, stop and make

a conscious choice about whether to keep eating it or not. This is the hardest one to do though!

The option you choose really depends on what suits you best, both at the time of the craving and in the longer term. However, the more often you can resist the craving (options 1 and 2), the more likely you are to 'reprogramme' your learned response to the culprit trigger, and the more likely it is that the craving will fade away. Again, the only way to see what works best is to practise different options. As a start, simply write your experiences in your food diary.

If you can't fend off a craving, see it as a learning experience. Plan how to deal with it differently next time, forgive yourself and move on. Don't let craving-based lapses push you off course – they're part of life. How you react to them could be more of a problem (see page 146).

Surfing and Distractions

One way of dealing with cravings is to 'surf' them. Imagine you are riding a wave that builds up, then crashes and ebbs away. Cravings are just like that and the longer you delay eating, the weaker the urge will become as a craving rarely lasts for more than 15 to 20 minutes. If it still hasn't gone by then, or if you need something else to do while 'surfing', distract yourself. Write a list of possible activities for when those difficult moments strike. Choose things you enjoy or get satisfaction from. The more active or involving the activity, the more effective it is. Here are some examples – and add some of your own ideas to the list.

- Phone or visit a friend
- Go out for a walk or cycle ride (without money or not near shops)
- Have a relaxing bath
- Visualize a wonderful holiday location
- Paint your nails

- Clean your teeth
- Do the ironing
- Work on a favourite task e.g. sewing, decorating, gardening

Do You Criticize Yourself a Lot?

When you look in the mirror do you say positive things – for example, that things are going very well overall and that half a stone has already made a difference? Or is it more like: 'I'll never be slim. I've only lost a measly half stone in four weeks. And I broke my diet last night. Typical! I may as well just give up.'

Both of these are examples of 'self-talk' – automatic thought or statements all of us constantly make to ourselves and which influence how we feel and act. Self-talk may be positive and constructive (like your guardian angel) or negative and irrational (like having a destructive devil perched on your shoulder).

If you've had on-off battles with your weight over the years, it's highly likely that it is the 'devil' who is there more often. Self-talk that says 'You're hopeless' can make you feel like a failure, which can then trigger you into the action of overeating and/or totally giving up. One of the worst things is that the latest thoughts we've had or words we've said are what stay in the mind. So if we think 'I still look fat' or 'I will never be slim' these are the thoughts that stay with us.

The trick is first to recognize that this is happening, then turn it around into a positive version of the same event – as in the first scenario above – so that the resulting action is to feel good and stay on track. Rather than being left with 'I still look fat' – keeping you focused on failure and your bad feelings about your appearance – you could be left with the positive 'I have lost half a stone which is great since I have had a lot on in the past two weeks' or 'I have accomplished many things in my life, so there is no reason why I can't manage my weight.'

Reshaping negative self-talk also helps to break or manage

destructive behaviour chains. And, most importantly, it helps you to change your self-definition, from someone who 'can't lose weight' or 'achieve this or that' to someone who 'can'. And when you believe you can – guess what happens.

Recognizing Negative Self-Talk

There are different types of negative or irrational self-talk that can make us our own harshest critics.

1 **Making definite demands** For example, using phrases like 'I must'; 'I will never'; I will always'. This assumes you can always do something a certain way, regardless. But in reality, it sets you up for failure as nothing can be that definite.

2 **Catastrophizing** You exaggerate a run-of-the-mill problem into a catastrophe. 'I only did 10 minutes on the treadmill last night rather than 20 minutes, which has ruined my whole week's efforts!'

3 **Disregarding good things** 'OK, so I've lost 2lbs this week, but next week it will be nothing, you'll see.'

4 **'All or nothing' thinking** 'I have eaten that chocolate and blown my diet, so I may as well give up now.'

5 **Over-generalization** 'I can't stand not being able to eat what I want.'

If you recognize any of these, tell the devil to get lost next time diet-breaking negative self-talk looms, and let in your guardian angel. He would say instead:

1 'My goal is to...'.; 'I will plan to...'.

2 'OK, I did less than planned, but I just wasn't feeling quite right. I'll be fine next time. This one short workout won't ruin my week's efforts.'

3 'It is good that I've lost 2 pounds this week, and even though I've lost confidence in my abilities in the past there's no real reason why I shouldn't lose another pound next week.'

4 'The chocolate bar won't ruin my diet, but if I think it has and keep on

eating my negative self-talk will ruin it. So I will get back on track.'

5   'I don't like having to eat differently from other people, but my weight-loss goals are very important to me, so I *can* stand it. After all, the world won't stop if I miss dessert, and I know I will feel great afterwards.'

Other things you can do

▪ Keep a positive achievement list. If you find that you often dwell on the negative, write down positive achievements every day. This could be to do with your eating or activity, or any aspect of your life – tidied your bedroom, mended your daughter's uniform, started reading a new book, spoke to your boss about holidays, did some weeding – anything! Start each day with a positive statement about yourself.

▪ Ask yourself what you might say to someone else who spoke or thought so negatively about themselves.

▪ Look for evidence 'for' and 'against' your irrational self-talk rather than just accepting it.

DEALING WITH DIET LAPSES

One diet lapse can lead to a relapse – and could then head for total collapse! But what is a lapse and, more importantly, how can you stop it happening again?

▪ A 'lapse' is a temporary slip-up or straying off track from your weight-loss plan. It could be overeating, or missing out on a regular exercise session.

▪ A 'relapse' is when you feel so guilty, fed up or hopeless that you abandon your weight loss plan.

▪ 'Collapse' is when you feel so hopeless you give up totally.

So how do you stop a lapse heading for collapse? First of all, appreciate that lapses are quite a normal and expected part of changing your eating and activity habits. A lapse isn't necessarily a problem in itself, but how you react to it could be. Rather than telling yourself off or feeling guilty, try to learn from the lapse. For example, how could you avoid lapsing again in a similar situation?

Remember, too, that one slip-up doesn't mean you have undone all your hard work so far. Put it behind you, get straight back on track and have your next planned meal or snack. Trying to compensate by skipping a meal can just make you hungry and more likely to lapse again.

Lapse Exercise

Think back to your last lapse and ask yourself what situations and/or feelings triggered it. Use this information to plan ways to improve your eating control and reduce the number of times you lapse in the future. And, most importantly, if (or should I say when) you do lapse again, don't collapse. Forgive yourself, get back on track and take comfort in the fact that there are ways you can deal with, and reduce the risk of, future lapses.

What if I am often truly hungry?

It can be a big problem if you often feel truly hungry when you are trying to eat differently to lose weight. One way to address this is by not going on a very low-calorie diet (unless it is medically advised) or a very rigid diet. What does help is having regular meals (see page 102) that include plenty of filling fruit and vegetables. Making protein-rich and low-GI carbohydrate-rich foods part of your meals also helps (see Step Three). Make sure you drink enough fluid, too.

Flexible Restraint

'Flexible restraint' is when you follow your eating plan or personal goals most of the time, but occasionally include favourite foods or have a meal out. It is opposed to 'rigid restraint', which involves strict and unbending dietary rules. Research suggests that flexible restraint is especially helpful for long-term weight control, whether this is to keep to a healthy weight, or maintain weight loss. As discussed in earlier chapters, successful slimmers develop a personal and flexible approach to eating, while those who tend to fail, and who put themselves at risk of eating problems such as bingeing, generally opt for rigid plans.

Flexible restraint greatly reduces the risk of 'all or nothing' thinking, relapsing and bingeing. It helps you to be satisfied by small amounts of your favourite foods, as you know you can eat them again at some point, rather than a particular occasion being your 'last chance'. It is a sign that you are in control of your food choices, and your weight. Flexible restraint is very much the essence of this book.

ENLIST ONGOING SUPPORT

Making long-lasting lifestyle changes affects not just the person making the changes, but also the people closest to them (keep this in mind if someone else in your family, or a friend is slimming and you are supporting them). The way they react to these changes can be a great help or hindrance to your progress. For example, you may decide to get more exercise by walking in the evening with the kids, but they can't think of anything worse. Or you like experimenting, but your husband hates vegetables and isn't prepared to forego his fry-ups – which tempt you. And who can stand it when well-meaning partners constantly say 'what are you doing eating that, you're meant to be on a diet?!'

Even people who usually like to do things by themselves find that some sort of ongoing support is helpful (including when they are maintaining their new weight). The same goes if you feel embarrassed about talking to other people about your weight, or don't want them to know you're losing weight. But there's no need to tell a lot of people. In fact, talking endlessly about what you are doing is usually unhelpful. The important thing is to find the kind of help that suits you best from something or someone you feel comfortable with. This could be a health professional, a book or magazine, a slimming chat room on the Internet or a slimming club. Or help could come from friends, family or work colleagues – or a combination of any of these.

Family or friends are one source of support, but some of them might feel that teasing or criticizing is the best way to goad you into action. The fact is, they aren't mind-readers and, unless you tell them what will be most helpful, they're unlikely to be able to support you no matter how hard they try.

Communication is vital. One way to encourage this is by writing down the things your family or friends do that are 'helpful' and also those that are 'less helpful'. Be quite specific. For example, a 'helpful' thing might be going for a walk with you in the evenings; a 'less helpful' thing might be regularly buying you chocolates as a reward. Why not write down the ways in which people can best support you?

BODY IMAGE

Body image is a term we often hear, but it isn't always clear what it means. Simply put, it is how we view our bodies – the picture we have in our mind of our size and shape and general appearance, and how we think and feel about them.

Unfortunately, it is very common for people to have a negative body image, especially if they are overweight. I suppose this is no big surprise, considering the 'slim is beautiful' culture we live in – sadly, a culture that doesn't seem to be about to change. Having a negative body image, or being 'dissatisfied' with your body, can be very upsetting. It can get in the way of making the healthy lifestyle changes you crave. It can increase the risk of binge eating and yo-yo dieting. It can also get to the very core of self-esteem (how much you like, accept and respect yourself as an overall person) and this can mean that you don't like yourself. And if you don't like yourself you may feel that you are incapable of making lifestyle changes, or that you are not worth making the effort for.

Of course, not everyone who is overweight has a negative body image, and not everyone who is dissatisfied with their body shape is affected by this. And, of course, not everybody wants to lose weight. But if you think that how you feel about your body stops you doing things you would like to do in life, including controlling your weight (or your binge eating or exercise avoidance), the following suggestions might help you.

Improving Your Body Image

Body image involves how we think and feel about our bodies. And from all that has been discussed in this section, you will know that how we think about things can influence just about everything! Negative self-talk can lead to a negative body image. If you ask someone how they view your body, what they see is likely to be very different to what you see. And it is possible to change how you view yourself.

We aren't born with a certain body image. It changes and develops as our bodies do. The young girl who didn't give her body much thought, and then goes through puberty with the changes it brings in breasts and body fat, may suddenly hate her body if she is desperate to stay slim like her new pop-video heroines.

Men or women who have long disliked their bodies and struggled with their weight can feel that this influences everything in their lives. If only they could lose weight they would be happier, more successful, have fewer problems, be a better person, and so on. (It may help to know that many slim people also have low self-esteem and concerns about their body image. While we may think they have 'nothing to worry about', they may too be distressed by certain aspects of their appearance and perceived lack of abilities). Remember, if 'the diet' is started with low self-esteem, its days are

Remember, if 'the diet' is started with low self-esteem, its days are numbered. The first slip-up, and negative self-talk will no doubt come pouring out. It's very hard to look after your needs properly, if you don't feel worthy. And if you are overweight, and have a negative body image, it can be difficult to like, respect and accept yourself.

Because realistic weight goals to improve your health mean that even when you have lost weight you still won't be as slim as fashion magazines say you should be, it can be easier to accept being a more realistic weight – if you like yourself and your body regardless.

Keep these points in mind, too.

- Challenging your negative thoughts and self-talk can be done and is worth the effort.
- Aim to separate self-esteem from body image. You are the sum of your parts, so explore and cherish them.
- Having a positive body image generally helps people to be more active.
- Remember that being very overweight is really a health issue.
- Keep your expectations about goal weights and rate of loss realistic, and remember that we all have different body shapes.
- Seek professional help if your feel that your body dissatisfaction is very distressing and stops you from achieving your desired changes.

Body Image Exercises

Have a look at these exercises. Some might seem quite difficult, so just do the best you can at first. But do try them again in the future. The more you challenge what you think about your body, and yourself, the better you will feel, and the more you will believe in yourself.

- List four things you like about yourself as an overall person.
- List four positive things about your body. Look in the mirror if you can.
- List four things a close friend might say they like about your appearance.
- Practise accepting (and believing) a compliment someone pays you.
- List four things you would like to do but have been putting them off

Taking Care of Yourself

Show yourself that you really do respect your body (and mind) by looking after it. Not just by nourishing and exercising it, but by giving it proper rest, relaxation and pleasure. Looking after yourself can be a help as you change how you eat, especially if 'head hunger' eating or comfort-eating meant you had coped better with day-to-day emotions and stresses. These small pleasures help replace what food gave you.

If your body image and self-esteem are poor you may think, and therefore feel, that you aren't worth looking after and so you spend your energy looking after everyone else. But you deserve time out, some pampering, a good night's sleep, or whatever it is that makes you feel, well, good. And if you feel good, you are more likely to feel and act positively, energetically and with belief in your abilities. You are also more likely to accept and enjoy compliments. Looking after yourself isn't being selfish. It is what you deserve, and will help you to achieve your goals.

Here are some ways in which people like to look after themselves. Tick the ones you do, or would like to try, and add any of your own.

- Having a long shower or bath, then moisturizing your body with lotion.
- Booking a massage or facial.
- Sitting down and reading your favourite magazine.
- Changing your hairstyle.
- Having an afternoon nap.
- Walking in the park and feeding the ducks.
- Going to the theatre or cinema.
- Gardening.
- Seeing a live band or going clubbing.
- Going to a yoga or t'ai chi class.
- Playing cards or a board game.
- Visiting a friend you haven't seen for a while.
- Watching a video with a good friend.

- Buying some new clothes – take a friend for fun and advice.
- Having a picnic.
- Applying a good-quality fake tan and/or experimenting with make-up.
- Going for a walk and a chat with one of your children, your partner or a close friend.
- Signing up for that evening class you've always wanted to do.

DISORDERED EATING

What Is Normal Eating?

When we are surrounded by an overload of information about diets and nutrition, or read what thin celebrities supposedly live on, it's easy to get confused about what 'normal' eating is. While there is no single correct way to eat, there are some guidelines that are most compatible with good health and a healthy relationship with food.

Normal eating is:

- Eating something at least three times a day
- Occasionally overeating or undereating
- Showing flexible restraint (see page 147)
- Deciding to eat less of the foods you like as you know you can eat them again another time
- Eating regularly and in a sufficient amount (and variety) to prevent an urge to binge eat
- Not always eating to lose weight but knowing that you can 'watch your weight'
- Not conveniently labelling yourself as 'vegetarian' or having a 'food intolerance' simply to avoid eating in front of others (this of course, doesn't refer to people who are vegetarian or have a true food intolerance)
- Knowing that eating well and looking after your body is important for good health, but also knowing that food is also about pleasure and that other things influence health too.

The Binge-Diet Cycle

For many people, bingeing or problems with overeating develop after frequent dieting. Breakfast might be skipped as you aim to stay at no more than 800 calories a day. Then it's cottage cheese and crackers for lunch – and two chocolate bars in the afternoon as you give in to hunger and preoccupation with food (eating too little or too rigidly just makes you think about food more). Eating 'too much' or a 'bad' food can cause feelings of failure, which can lead to a blowout. The classic deprivation – binge cycle is in motion. In extreme cases, this cycle can contribute to recognized eating disorders such as bulimia nervosa or binge-eating disorder. But more commonly, this lurching between overeating and undereating causes distress and doesn't help people to control their weight safely or effectively.

Low self-esteem,
feel fat, bad,
a failure, guilty

Start a diet
Set rigid 'bad' food/
'good' food rules

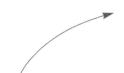

May overeat even more
Overeat, eat a
'bad' food, binge

Feel hungry, deprived,
fed up, bored, depressed

Do You Have a Problem with Binge-Eating?

We all overeat at times – and no doubt many of us overeat more often than we would like to. It's easy to describe overeating as having 'a binge'. But 'a binge' can mean different things to different people. For some it may be having a three-course meal – followed by a bit of guilt; while for others it could be a 'spaced out' hour-long assault on the fridge and cupboards followed by crippling self-loathing. So when does simple overeating become a more problematic binge? And what can you do if it gets out of control?

A binge is an eating occasion with both of these characteristics.

- Eating an amount of food that is excessively larger than an amount people would 'normally' eat in a similar situation, within a certain time period (say two hours)
- Feeling out of control during the eating period.

It is this feeling of 'a lack of control' that really distinguishes a binge from overeating. Even then, some people may have a true binge from time to time without it being a real problem. But others binge frequently, to the extent that it seriously affects their lives. This is known as 'binge-eating disorder' (see page 156). Step Four gives guidance on how to manage overeating, and better recognize the triggers that lie behind it.

What Helps People to Break Free from the Binge–Diet Cycle

Research shows that help can come from cognitive behavioural therapy (see page 54) techniques such as structured meal plans based on regular meals and snacks, keeping a diary to record food intake, thoughts and binges, and becoming armed with skills and strategies for recognizing and dealing with problem triggers and negative self-talk (see page 145). If people are overweight (not everyone with binge-eating problems is), it is usually helpful to first try to stabilize eating patterns and reduce or stop bingeing, rather than keep trying to lose weight. If you ever find yourself on the verge (or in the middle) of a binge, these strategies can help:

- Stop doing whatever you are doing, and move away from the situation. For example, walk out of the kitchen.
- Stay calm and congratulate yourself on stopping the binge.
- If you still feel like bingeing, imagine how you would feel after the binge, and compare that to how you would feel if you stopped now.
- Use the situation to work out which triggers led to the binge.
- Do something else to distract you from the situation.
- Have your next meal as usual, and stay positive; don't tell yourself off.
- Reflect on how you could avoid a similar situation in the future.

If you find controlling your eating too difficult to manage by yourself, do talk to your doctor who may be able to refer you to a state-registered dietitian or clinical psychologist.

EATING DISORDERS

Eating disorders such as anorexia nervosa, bulimia nervosa and binge-eating disorder are very serious and develop as outward signs of inner emotional problems or psychological distress. People use bingeing, or restricting food intake, to help them cope with difficulties and low self-worth. Sufferers have a distorted body image and their lives are governed by weight and shape concerns. While eating disorders can affect people of almost any age, the peak age of onset for anorexia nervosa is 16 to 18 years – when up to one per cent of girls may suffer from the disorder – with a smaller peak at the time of puberty. Bulimia nervosa is most common amongst 18 to 25-year-olds, and is thought to affect 1–2 per cent of women. But these are not just female problems. Approximately one in ten of all people with eating disorders are men. People with eating disorders need specialist help.

Because we live in a society that exerts great pressure to be slim, dieting and body dissatisfaction have long been seen as causes of eating disorders. For this reason, there is concern that encouraging people to control their weight could lead to disordered eating patterns, especially amongst young people. Studies certainly suggest that obesity in childhood, or repeated dieting during adolescence, increases risk, but body dissatisfaction and its effect in lowering self-esteem may be the more fundamental problem. It's important to remember that true eating disorders are very complex conditions and are not about dieting going too far. The vast majority of people who diet don't have eating disorders. However, a proportion of children, teenagers and adults do have problems with food – comfort-eating, bingeing, skipping meals and occasional laxative abuse – that could be detrimental to their weight, nutritional health and emotional well-being. As parents, partners and health professionals we must always be mindful of this. But we must also be mindful of the negative health effects of obesity. Promoting healthy and realistic messages about weight control, and nurturing a positive body image and self-esteem, seems the best way forward.

Night-eating Syndrome

People with 'night-eating syndrome' complain of eating large amounts of food at night, often without fully realizing what they are doing. They then try to compensate by eating less during the day. Night-eating is thought to be a response to stress and anxiety, but it is not clear whether it is a sleep disorder or an eating disorder.

Helping Children Develop Healthy Attitudes to Food and Weight

The rise in overweight and obese people of all ages and the fact that eating disorders are also very real and very worrying illnesses, means there is understandable concern about how best to help our children.

Children's eating habits, exercise habits and body image can be influenced by their parents' habits, and by early experiences. Babies are born with a liking for sweet tastes, and rapidly take to fatty and salty ones, but need to learn to like everything else. So is it any wonder that a young child living in an environment where there are plenty of opportunities to eat crisps and biscuits goes for them rather than greens! It is even more difficult if less popular foods are presented in a negative way – 'Eat your vegetables, or you won't be able to play with Jimmy tomorrow.' Or if they are taken off the menu after a first refusal – repeated offering does increase acceptance.

Studies also show that children who eat regular meals with their family eat more fruit and vegetables, and eat less fat in food, both at home and away from home. Similar results have been found if families eat at a table as opposed to in front of the television. Watching less television also helps to prevent obesity in children.

Parental attitudes to food and their own weight can also influence children's body image and eating habits. Research from Pennsylvania State University found that three- to six-year-old girls with mothers who ate whether they were hungry or not when offered good-tasting food, were also most likely to carry on eating when full – and to be overweight.

Children are very good mimics, so mothers influenced by magazine images and the general 'slim is beautiful' culture may, albeit unwittingly, pass their weight and shape concerns on to their children. The same Pennsylvania State University research found that five-year-old girls are weight conscious because their mothers are on diets. This mirrors research in the UK which found links between the way ten-year-old girls talk about restricting their food because of weight concerns and their mothers' comments about food and weight. There has been little research with fathers, but they should be aware of their potential to make thoughtless comments about their child's appearance. The same goes for teasing taunts from siblings.

Inactive parents generally have inactive children, and studies indicate that parents who want to influence their children's inactivity need to lead by example, as well as offering encouragement and support. To help our children it seems we must first look to our own lifestyle habits and body images.

So What Can Parents Do?

Because we live in a toxic environment just about all of us, including children, need to show some sort of dietary restraint and planned increase in activity to keep to a healthy weight. Past research suggested that dietary restraint and dieting led to overeating, but research is now suggesting that 'flexible restraint' (see page 147) can be beneficial. It is 'rigid restraint', involving strict dietary rules and forbidden foods, that is potentially problematic and may increase the risk of eating disorders.

Food can be a powerful tool for children to wind their parents up with, or to express their individualism – a bit like new fashions. It may be tempting to respond to this by exerting more control over what they do, or bottling up anxiety – but this frequently leads to a battle. However, it can help if parents understand why their children are behaving in a certain way – and keep the lines of communication open. The same goes for trying to encourage more activity – for example, by putting a limit on watching television. Negotiation, rather than just telling children what to do, is the key.

If children do have a weight problem parents are often concerned that any attempt to help may trigger an eating disorder. However, there is currently no real evidence to support this view, especially if the whole family also makes changes. Guiding your children towards healthy food choices and active lifestyles is a positive and caring thing to do. As parents you can only help in the best ways possible and support your child regardless of his or her body shape. When parents help an overweight child to eat a balanced diet, with occasional treats, the child actually ends up eating well and has the healthiest diet. Surely it makes sense for everyone in the family to eat this way?

Tips for Parents

- Be a good role model – it will also help your health and weight.
- Make sure you have a good knowledge of what a healthy diet is, and how to be more active.
- Examine your own feelings about weight and body shape.
- Talk to your children about how things are at school, how they feel about themselves, their friends, anything that is going on.
- Find something your child really enjoys and is good at.
- Help your children to recognize their self-worth in terms of things that they do or say, not their appearance.
- Talk through the health benefits of being more active and eating healthily – rather than 'appearance' benefits.
- Help your children to recognize when they feel physically hungry and when they are satisfied.
- Help your children to develop natural feelings of hunger and fullness by ensuring regular balanced meals, not making them clear their entire plate if they have almost finished; having, say, fruit or yogurt in easy reach for snacks, and keeping treat-like snacks behind cupboard doors.
- Recognize that there is no ideal body shape, and that we are all different shapes and sizes.
- Ensure your children understand how their bodies will change as they grow older and develop.
- If weight problems run in your family, perhaps explain the link between genes and environment, and how your family has to take care but will be healthier for it.
- Be positive and supportive, rather than negative and closed to negotiation.
- Keep special foods for special occasions rather than for everyday eating.
- Eat together whenever you can and involve your children in food

preparation; food is social and pleasurable as well as nourishing.

- Ensure that the whole family is encouraged to follow the same flexible healthy behaviours, rather than singling one child out.
- Get involved with improving school meals/food provision at school.
- Try not to let food become a power struggle, nor a means of reward or punishment.
- If you have real concerns about a child's weight, or eating behaviour, see your doctor. He or she can advise you directly or let you know about local specialist services.

step five

energize your daily life

LET'S GET PHYSICAL!

Food is one side of the energy equation. Now to have fun with the other side: physical activity. While we all know that exercise is good for us, the importance of just moving more each day has been relatively overlooked. In fact, being more active is proven to be one of the most effective ways to control your weight for good. And many of us, me included until recently, don't appreciate the extent to which being active helps both our physical and our mental health. Being active also isn't just about doing some sort of 'exercise'. It's about moving more, more often and seeing every opportunity to move as being a positive way to help you be fitter and slimmer.

Being inactive doubles your risk of dying from any cause, and is the key factor behind more than a third of all deaths from heart disease in the UK. This makes physical activity at least as important as not smoking and eating a healthy diet. It is also estimated that half of all hip fractures could be avoided with regular physical activity.

Here's a run-through of the many reasons why being active is so vital for our overall well-being. Regular physical activity helps to:

- Prevent and treat overweight and obesity
- Preserve muscle strength (and metabolism) when weight is lost
- Regulate appetite
- Maintain a healthier weight after weight loss
- Reduce high blood pressure
- Lower risk of heart disease and stroke
- Lower blood triglycerides and raise 'good' HDL cholesterol
- Reduce the risk of colon cancer, and possibly breast cancer

- Reduce the risk of osteoporosis (brittle bones)
- Reduce the risk of type 2 diabetes
- Treat diabetes
- Raise self-esteem and self-efficacy (belief in your abilities)
- Improve mood and prevent depression
- Allow better sleep
- Manage stress and anxiety
- Increase stamina and flexibility
- Prevent low back pain

How Does Activity Help Our Weight?

In Section One we discussed energy balance and how our weight is a balance between the calories we consume and the calories we burn or expend. Physical activity is a key contributor to the 'calories expended' side of the balance – it's also the part we have most control over. If we expend more calories than we consume we will lose weight. Physical activity helps us to do that in a number of ways. It really is a win-win situation.

- Our metabolic rate is increased by activity and encourages the body to burn fat.
- Regular physical activity helps to build muscle and counteract muscle loss that normally comes with weight loss, so off-setting falls in your metabolic rate.
- In 24 hours 0.45kg (1lb) of body fat burns around two calories while 0.45kg (1lb) of muscle burns around 35 calories, so you want to hang on to what muscle you can!
- It helps us to feel more confident and in control of our weight, which makes it easier to achieve realistic and sustainable goals.

Physical activity helps our weight most when it is combined with dietary change. As you will see in the table on page 173–4, you need to be active for long periods to burn enough calories to have a big impact on weight loss in the short term. For example, to lose 0.25kg

(½lb) a week through exercise alone you would need to do a 45-minute walk every day. By diet – this can be done by cutting 250 calories from your current calorie needs – say, a chocolate bar, each day. This is OK, but if you did both you could lose closer to 0.45kg (1lb) a week, optimize muscle strength and boost your general health and well-being. Physical activity's greatest benefits for weight control are over the longer term. For example, adding a daily 30-minute brisk walk could lead to a 5.5kg (12lb) weight loss over a year.

Regular physical activity has an even stronger impact on maintaining weight loss. This is great news, since keeping the weight off is usually the hardest part. More good news is that being active also counteracts what can seem like inevitable middle-aged weight gain.

People are often put off the idea of being more active because they think it means being sporty and having to run around parks or work out in gyms. If you are very overweight, this is a further deterrent because you may find it physically difficult to be active, or feel uncomfortable about exercising in public. The good news here is that being more active doesn't mean you have to go near a gym or aerobics class if you don't want to. In fact, research suggests that keeping up moderate activity (see below) is the most effective way of controlling weight.

All this is well and good but, like any change in behaviour, you have to be motivated to do it for yourself, and you must feel that the potential benefits outweigh the potential downsides. We talked about this in Step One, but it makes sense to take another look specifically in connection with activity.

Changing your activity levels takes the same sort of commitment as changing your eating habits – although some people may find one more straightforward than the other. It means having to change your usual routine, finding time to fit something else into your day, and confronting body-image concerns that may have held you back from being more active in the past. All the skills about SMART goal-setting, coping with lapses (missed exercise rather than too many cream cakes this time!), positive self-talk, rewarding your achievements and staying motivated are as relevant to physical activity as they are to eating. If you haven't prepared yourself properly, again it's very easy to slip at the first hurdle, or simply feel that it's not worth the effort. That would be a great pity because all the research screams out that being more active, and staying that way, is one of the best indicators of long-term slimming success.

Have a heart for activity

Men and women who are physically active have around half the risk of having a heart attack compared to people who are inactive. Being active helps our heart work better by keeping the heart muscle strong, giving it a good oxygen supply, keeping its arteries flexible, lowering blood pressure, optimizing blood fats and reducing the risk of blood clots.

Take a few moments to think about and write down the pros and cons of being more active. Remember to also think in terms of the consequences of each – that is, what the outcome of being more active, or not, will be and what might you have to forego. If you find there are more pros than cons you should feel highly motivated to be more active. If you aren't sure, it's worth giving more physical activity a go to see how you find it. So keep reading. You may find that being more active is not as complicated as you think. And, as you know, how we think about things affects how we feel and act.

PROS OF BEING MORE ACTIVE	CONS OF BEING MORE ACTIVE
Will make me feel more alive, help me lose weight	Hate feeling sweaty, need to find time
Will keep me away from the kitchen after work	Will mean I have less time for some other things

How Active Should We Be?

Eighty per cent of adults think they are physically active. But statistics show that we are far too optimistic. According to the British Heart Foundation, only about 25 per cent of women and 37 per cent of men are active enough to benefit their health. The older we get the less active and fitter we are, too. For example, most women over 35 and men over 55 are not able to walk up a moderate slope at a normal pace without getting breathless and having to stop to avoid feeling uncomfortably 'puffed'. Our children are also much less active than they used to be. About 40 per cent of boys and 60 per cent of girls fail to spend an average of one hour a day in activities – the recommended guideline for young people.

UK health and fitness experts recommend the following as the minimum level of physical activity that will benefit our health:

▪ Accumulate 30 minutes of moderate intensity activity on at least five days a week. 'Moderate intensity' activity is equivalent to brisk walking, or an activity such as gardening, cycling, dancing, swimming, tennis or heavy housework like vacuuming and scrubbing that makes you feel warm and breathe more heavily than usual. To ensure you aren't over-exerting yourself, you should still be able to have a conversation (it's fine to feel a bit breathless) while you are doing the activity. If you can hardly speak at all, slow down!

Boost your self-esteem

Being more active helps our well-being in many ways. In fact, studies suggest that it raises self-esteem in both adults and children (which helps confidence and body image), as well as relieving symptoms of depression, anxiety and low mood. It also makes depression less likely to develop in the first place.

Moderate means maintenance

A number of studies have highlighted how being moderately active for 30 minutes or so every day can be just as good for our health as going to the gym a few times a week. Those who intermittently go 'for the burn' are also at risk of being couch potatoes in between, or they may eat too much as a reward for being active (it only takes a few minutes to consume the calories burned by an hour's workout) and end up back at square one – if not minus one! This is heartening news because many people simply don't like the idea of, or can't afford, gym visits (but if you do like them, they can be a valuable part of being more active overall). However, simply being more active every day can be enough to make a difference. For example, one participant in a study, who was doing nothing before, enjoyably and painlessly built in her 30 minutes of extra walking by doing day-to-day things like parking further away from the shops, using stairs and walking around the house during TV commercials. Now it's just a habit for her.

- The fact that activity can be accumulated means you can do 10-or 15-minute sessions over the day if you can't manage the 30 minutes at one time. And the exercise can be made up of a variety of moderately intense activities you enjoy if you don't want to just stick to one.
- If you haven't exercised for some time, you will need to build up gradually over a few weeks. It also helps if you can build more general activity into your daily routine.

When you are losing weight, aiming to burn at least 1000 calories and, if possible, up to 2000 calories a week through extra activity is ideal. On average, this amounts to 30 to 60 minutes of brisk walking each day. But, as for all goals, it is vital to work out what is realistic for you and go from there. Remember, 30 minutes at least five days a week is enough to improve well-being and fitness, and moving more, more often helps to manage your weight.

Why Are We So Inactive?

What is often described as a 'sedentary lifestyle' means mostly sitting, or doing light activities such as moving about home and work as you get on with the basic needs of daily living. Thanks to our toxic environment – and the way it encourages us to drive cars from A to B, take lifts rather than stairs, sit and watch TV or PCs, and push buttons to light fires, wash clothes and even do the shopping (via the Internet) – we can live our lives doing very little indeed. These days we demand convenience. But this just means we expend even less effort and energy getting things done. To overcome this we need to replace sedentary daily activities with more active ones e.g. replacing 30 minutes of TV with a walk, or taking the stairs rather than the escalator.

Of course, some people are not physically able to be active, or are limited in what they can do for health reasons. If this applies to you, do speak to your doctor. He or she may be able to advise you directly on what activities may be suitable, or refer you for specialist advice. You may still find some of the information in this section helpful – for example, you may be able to manage arm exercises, or a gentle walking programme (see page 176).

What Is Physical Activity?

Physical activity refers to all energy expended by movement. This includes daily living activities such as walking, climbing stairs and gardening. Exercise is physical activity that is intentional and aims to improve some aspect of fitness or health. Of course, many people participate in exercise for pleasure and the challenge of competitive sport. Exercise can include regular walking but can also mean aerobics, martial arts, weight training, and a variety of sports. Active pastimes such as gardening or dancing are also 'exercise' if they are planned and carried out for long enough to enhance health and well-being.

One simple way to motivate yourself to be more active every day, and have a bit of fun at the same time, is to use a pedometer. These battery-operated gadgets are simply clipped on to your belt or waistband, and let you know how many steps you take each day. Some even play music and talk to you about your progress! They currently cost about £10–£15 and can be bought at popular sports shops. To help your health, and your weight, the aim is to take 10,000 steps daily – more if you can. If you don't walk much at the moment it could take a couple of weeks or so to build up to that. Remember, any increase in the amount you move is progress. But to achieve long-lasting change, it helps to have some clear, yet sustainable, goals to help you get results.

Different Types of Activity

Physical activity can be separated into different types, but all can be used to help you move more – more often. It's really about doing whatever you enjoy most and whatever is simplest to fit into your routine. Many people find that they once they get going they use a combination of a few of the types of activity listed below, especially doing more routine and spontaneous activities. The '30 minutes of moderate intensity activity on at least five days a week' message helps the fitness of our heart and lungs, our metabolism (insulin and blood fat levels) and our muscle and bone strength.

These are the main types of physical activity.

Routine Walking to shops; walking the dog; gardening; climbing stairs at home; housework; making the bed; cooking; shopping; bathing; a regular hobby.

Spontaneous Looking for ways to replace being sedentary with activity. For example, using the stairs rather than the lift; gardening; getting off the bus one stop earlier and walking further; DIY;

switching off the TV and doing something else.

Continuous Aerobic Activity Planned exercise that gets the heart and lungs working. For example, cycling; taking a brisk walk; swimming; line-dancing; rowing which get the heart and lungs working.

Structured Organized sport or leisure-time activity. For example, football; netball; tennis; golf; hiking; bowling.

Muscle Toning Exercise that especially stretches, tones or builds the muscles (also called resistance training). For example, yoga; weights; circuit training; toning classes.

How to Exercise Without Doing Anything

Don't be fooled by this one! It's like all those weight-loss potions and quick-fix diets that promise painless, rapid weight loss while you eat what you like – whether it's 'spot reducing' treatments, saunas to make you sweat, gadgets to make your muscles twitch or tables that move your legs for you. They might sound great but they won't help you get fitter or burn more calories like real activity does – unless you get very agitated when you see the cost of some of them!

Barriers to Being More Active

Things often get in the way of the best intentions, or you might be motivated to be more active but just can't get your head around some of the barriers that present themselves to you. You aren't alone here, but 'Where there's a will there's a way', and part of your physical activity skill development is using SMART goals to use your 'will skill' to find a way around barriers. Successful slimmers think positive and believe they can do it. They don't just talk about the fact they are going to join a gym, or go for a walk every morning; they get up and go. But first they work out how to overcome their potential barriers.

Here's what other people have said are common barriers. Do any sound familiar to you? Add others that specifically affect you to the list.

- Lack of time due to other commitments, such as work, family.
- Can't afford to spend money on it.
- Not knowledgeable about the sort of activities that benefit health.
- Not a 'sporty' type; don't know how to play sports or work out.
- Lack motivation or willpower.
- Will make me want to eat more.
- Simply too lazy.
- Lack someone to exercise with me or encourage me.
- Not very welcoming at clubs.
- Lack of babysitting facilities.
- Don't enjoy it; don't like feeling sweaty and puffed out.
- Worried about overdoing it or straining something.
- Self-conscious about being active in front of others.
- Find it uncomfortable because of weight.

Make a list of some of your own barriers.

But I can't exercise because...

'I am worried about injuring myself or looking foolish. I also can't afford a health club'.

Reply: 'Walking is the safest activity. It is also straightforward, cheap and something you can fit into your routine. Start slowly and build up.'

'I don't have anyone to be active with – so I won't do it.'

Reply: 'Check out what's on locally and whether there are any community schemes, such as health walks, environmentally focused initiatives or exercise referral schemes. Ask at your library, doctor's surgery or local sports centre, or look in the Yellow Pages. Many adult education or evening classes cover exercise-based subjects, such as martial arts, aerobics or different types of dancing. This could be the time to learn flamenco, get to grips with self-defence, play netball again or learn to scuba dive (starting in the pool)!'

'I am worried that it will make me eat more'.

Reply: 'The good news is that a number of studies now show that a moderate level of exercise doesn't make you hungrier or drive the body to eat more to compensate for the calories burned by physical activity. If anything, exercise helps you to regulate your appetite better. It can also make you feel better about yourself, which in turn helps people feel positive about eating wisely. However, it's not all good news. Some people overestimate the calories burned by exercise or feel they need to "reward" themselves with high-calorie treats. This can mean they end up eating more calories than they burned and so slowly gain weight, when they think they should be losing it!'

'I don't have enough time to fit it in'.

Reply: 'Find ways that you can fit in more opportunistic "spontaneous" activity. For example, at home and at work use the toilet on the next floor up/in furthest part of the house (unless desperate!); take a 15-minute walk at lunchtime rather than sitting; put out your walking shoes and tracksuit so that they are there to slip on when you first get up in the morning for a 15-minute walk – take your personal stereo and listen to the morning news. At the supermarket, park as far away from the main doors as you can. The time spent walking there and back will be saved by the ease of parking.'

Calories Burned by Different Activities

The time (in minutes) that you need to spend at a certain activity in order to burn either 150 or 250 calories is shown below. The values are based on the calories that would be burned by a 76kg (12 stone) person. Lighter people would burn slightly fewer calories, and heavier people slightly more, doing the same activity. The more intense the activity, the more calories expended, but you can mix and match activities to help you be more active and achieve your daily goals.

Activity	150 calories	250 calories
Aerobics (medium intensity)	20 minutes	33 minutes
Aerobics (high intensity)	14	23
Badminton	20	33
Card playing	80	133
Cleaning	31	52
Cycling (leisurely)	31	52
Cycling (moderately)	20	33
Dancing (modern)	20	33
Dancing (ballroom)	38	63
Gardening (digging)	15	25
Gardening (raking)	35	58
Golf	23	38
Horse-riding (trotting)	18	30
Ironing	60	100
Judo	10	17
Painting (inside)	58	97
Running – slow (11-minute mile)	14	23
Running – rapid (7-minute mile)	10	17
Scrubbing floors	18	30
Sitting quietly/TV watching	95	158
Skipping	12	20
Squash	9	15
Standing	75	125
Swimming (breaststroke)	12	20
Swimming (freestyle, slow)	16	37
Table tennis	29	58
Tennis	18	30

Walking (average pace)	33	55
Walking (briskly)	25	42
Walking uphill	15	25
Window cleaning	33	55

SETTING GOALS AND MONITORING PROGRESS

Setting personal goals that are achievable and sustainable is the key to long-term weight-control success. This is especially important if you have had bad experiences with exercise programmes in the past and have been put off. It can be hard to know what is safe, and effective. As with changing your eating habits, taking things slowly, developing skills and getting help and support will really help.

Keeping a written record of your goals and your progress each day is very motivating. As with your food diary, it is also useful for looking back to see how things have changed over time, and it will remind you to stay aware of fitting in more activity. This is all part of taking care of yourself, and can be a truly enjoyable and motivating experience.

Think about some activities that you feel you could realistically fit into your day-to-day life. Are they also things you will enjoy enough to keep them up long term? Write them down. Now choose one and develop SMART goals to help you achieve it (see page 56).

S = Specific

M = Measurable

A = Achieveable

R = Realistic

T = Time-specific

For example, your chosen goal may be to build up a walking programme as on page 176. This has specific and measurable aspects – and you can record your week-by-week progress in your food diary. Also write down where and when you will walk, whether you need to walk with anyone else and, if so, who, and whether you need anything special – say, a good pair of walking shoes. Write down when you will get your walking shoes. Make a note, too, of any time you do any other type of intentional activity, such as using the stairs when you would have once used the lift. It all adds up and it all feels good.

Once you start your walking programme, think about how you feel at the end of each week. See how that matches up to some of the pros of being more active that you thought about earlier. If you are having trouble staying positive, or have missed some days of walking and feel ready to give up – read Step Four again. A slip-up or two won't ruin your efforts, so think positive, stay on track and plan how you can avoid a similar slip-up in the future.

Tried and Trusted Tips

- Get into a regular routine by being active at a similar time each day.
- Plan ahead, especially if your usual routine is about to change – for example if you go away; the weather changes; you need to do something different with the family.
- Choose an activity you enjoy. If you find that difficult, make it part of something you have to do anyway, such as walking the dog, doing the shopping or the housework – find ways to walk more, and more briskly, and put more effort into those chores.
- Walk up and down escalators and always take the stairs rather than the lift. (If there are a lot of flights, take the lift part of the way.)
- Use an exercise bike in front of the television or listen to the radio or music as you walk.
- Make an activity date with a friend, or take up an activity that involves other people – this will help you to keep up your commitment.

Get Ready, Get Set, Go

It is always wise to start exercise carefully. If you haven't exercised for a long time and are over 50, or if you are very overweight and/or have another medical problem such as diabetes, high blood pressure or a heart condition, it's wise to check with your doctor before you start any activity programme. Ensure that you have some comfortable clothes, and good supportive footwear. Seek advice from a sports shop if you aren't sure.

The different types of activities you can choose from, and the optimal amount of exercise you need to take each day to get you fitter and healthier has been discussed. So has the importance of not pushing yourself too hard to start with – you should be able to hold a conversation while you're at it!

While there are many regular activities you could do, such as cycling or swimming, Dr David Ashton, Director of the Healthier Weight Centre in Birmingham, and an exercise expert, is a strong advocate of walking, especially for people who are losing weight (and keeping it off).

If you haven't exercised for a while, your doctor has advised a gradual start to activity or you would like a more structured approach to being active, Dr Ashton recommends the following walking programme.

Walking Programme

Warm Up and Cool Down

Before and after walking (or any other aerobic or sporting activity), it's a good idea to do some gentle stretching exercises. For example:

- **Side reaches** Reach one arm over your head and to the side. Keep your hips steady and your shoulders straight to the side. Hold for 10 seconds and repeat on the other side.
- **Knee pull** Lean your back against a wall. Keep your head, hips and feet in a straight line. Pull one knee to your chest, hold for 10 seconds, then repeat with the other leg.
- **Leg curl** Pull your foot to your buttocks with your opposite hand. Keep your knee pointing straight to the ground. Hold for 10 seconds and repeat with the other hand.

When you begin walking, make sure you:

- Walk with your chin up and your shoulders held slightly back.
- Wear comfortable footwear with good ankle support.
- Walk so that the heel of your foot touches the ground first, then roll your weight forward.
- Walk with your toes pointed forward and swing your arms as you walk.
- Stop if you feel dizzy, very tired or unwell, or experience any pain.

Aim to do the following on at least five days a week – every day if you can.

Week	Warm up Walk slowly for (minutes)	Fast walk Walk briskly for (minutes)	Cool down Walk slowly for (minutes)	Total time (minutes)
One	5	5	5	15
Two	5	7	5	17
Three	5	9	5	19
Four	5	11	5	21
Five	5	13	5	23
Six	5	15	5	25
Seven	5	18	5	28
Eight	5	20	5	30
Nine	5	23	5	33
Ten	5	26	5	36
Eleven	5	28	5	38
Twelve	5	30	5	40

For Week Thirteen and beyond, gradually increase your brisk walking time from 30 to 60 minutes, five or more days a week.

Resistance Training

Don't overlook the benefits of gentle weight or resistance training. While it is not as big a calorie burner as aerobic activities like walking or cycling, it does help to slow down or reverse the loss of muscle size and strength that comes with age and, to a certain extent, with weight loss. Resistance training also helps bone strength, co-ordination, flexibility and general well-being. This makes it an ideal complement to aerobic activities like regular walking. Again, it is wise to speak to your doctor before weight training – and essential if you have a medical problem. It's important to know how to use weights properly, so seek advice from a gym or health club before you start. Building up to 20–30 minutes, two to three times a week is an ideal target, but whatever you can manage on a regular basis will help. You can buy weights for home use – once you know what you're doing. If you ever feel unwell while training, stop immediately.

FAMILY ACTIVITY

If you are a parent, grandparent or care for children, there's nothing like being a good role model and encouraging active family living. Here are some ideas to talk to your children about:

- Walk or ride to school – with older children or parents if you are concerned about safety.
- Join in active games at school or at a sports, exercise or youth club.
- Use stairs rather than lifts and escalators.
- Walk the dog with you – or pretend to if you don't have one!
- Help with active jobs around the house and garden.
- Limit computer and TV time.
- Buy toys that promote physical activity – such as balls, sports games.
- Develop active family pursuits – dancing, bike-riding, rollerblading.

step six

taking care of yourself, and your family, for life

LOOK TO THE FUTURE

By now you will have got the picture that *Diet Trials* is not just a guide to losing weight quickly. It is about acquiring the skills, confidence and ongoing motivation to help you to achieve a healthier weight. And while you are doing that, the same skills will be preparing you to maintain that healthier weight once the major 'change' period is over –or will help you to keep to your current weight.

I am not suddenly going to pretend that it's easy to maintain a healthy weight. The statistics wouldn't support me even if I tried. The fact is that long-term studies show that most people who lose a significant amount of weight have put much of it back on after three to five years. But not everyone does, and more people seem to be getting better at managing their weight long-term – especially those who follow the sort of advice in this book.

The most important thing to realize is that once you've lost weight, if you go back to the old habits that caused you to be overweight in the first place – how you ate, how active (or inactive) you were, how you thought and felt about yourself – your weight will come back on. And I imagine that you have been there too many times before – or don't want to start such a destructive cycle. To look after yourself you need to stay conscious of, and responsible for, your lifestyle. There is no way around this. Other people can help and support you – this is vital, especially if you are very overweight or have struggled with your weight for a long time, but ultimately you have to do it yourself. Remember the saying – 'If you do what you have always done, you will get what you have always got.' Thanks to your new skills, confidence and attitude, you have the power to change and to get what you want.

Fortunately, many old unhelpful habits will now be replaced by new, helpful ones. But remember, you are still in the toxic environment and, like everyone else, you have a body designed to eat in the midst of plenty (in case that plenty disappears). It is an environment that your genes may be particularly unsuited for, meaning that you have to work that bit harder than some people. An environment that seductively entices you to overeat and be inactive. Yes, you will let yourself be seduced by it now and then, but it won't get the better of you and indulgences are likely to be planned. This is the skill of flexible restraint.

You are the one in control here, not the environment or your genetic make-up. And while you can't control the environment itself, you can control how you deal with it. You have your 'head straight'. You appreciate what is realistic for you. You know what you want, you believe you can do it, you feel that you are worth doing it for and you make conscious choices to achieve it. You stay aware of your eating and activity habits – and any negative self-talk that hovers around the edges. If you find yourself wavering, you forgive yourself, then remind yourself of the importance of staying at a healthier weight. You are sacrificing a little for enormous benefits. A healthier, nurtured body, mind and soul – and the knowledge that you may have given yourself another nine years to get the best from life.

Keeping the Balance Right After Weight Loss

If you have lost weight and now want to stabilize at your new healthier weight, you need to get into energy balance – where the calories you consume are in balance with the energy you burn.

After losing a realistic 5 to 10 per cent of your weight, you may be happy with what you weigh now and want to maintain this longterm. Or if you were very overweight to start with, and would like to lose more weight for your health's sake, it can help if you spend some time getting used to living at your new weight before moving on to lose some more. Research shows that people often find it difficult to keep losing weight for more than about 12 weeks at a time. What you decide to do is, of course, up to you. It is worth remembering though, research also suggests that people who remain realistic about their ultimate goal weight are the ones who are most likely to reach them and stay there – in contrast to those who aspire, or even get, to a lower 'dream' weight then pile it all back on.

Because you haven't been following quick-fix diet plans or extreme exercise programmes, but have been making personal and sustainable lifestyle changes, what you do next shouldn't involve any dramatic changes.

If you decide to keep losing weight gradually, and have been making changes for three months or so, you may need to review your goals, including your eating and activity plans. Do keep up your food (and activity diary), or some form of self-monitoring, even if it's only for three or four days a week. Studies show that people who continue to self-monitor at least 50 per cent of the time continue to make changes and lose weight.

If you are ready to maintain your weight – or your aim all along has been to maintain it (rather than slowly gain) – again it is really a matter of keeping up and reinforcing your new skills, attitudes and outlook. If you go back to past habits extra weight will come back on. If your weight had already stabilized naturally there is nothing to change. If you had been losing around 0.45kg (1lb) a week until the time you decided to stabilize, you can eat a bit more – typically around 200 to 300 calories or so. Keep up your regular meals, and the sorts of foods you would normally choose, but have, say, a slightly bigger breakfast or evening meal, or an extra snack. Or it might all come out in the wash and you will find that you can eat out or enjoy favourite foods a bit more often. Remember to practise flexible restraint.

When it comes to activity, aim to keep more or less to what you have been doing. If you have been regularly working out each week in addition to taking a daily 30 minute walk, for example, you could taper down the workouts if you like. The key thing is to keep up that daily (or most days) 'moderate intensity' activity as a lifelong habit, along with more active leisure time like a long walk in the park. The research is particularly strong about the impact staying active has on maintaining weight loss – and preventing weight gain in the first place.

Some trial and error can be involved in getting the balance established. Keep a regular check (say, weekly or fortnightly) on your weight (or waist measurement, or how your fitted clothes feel) and aim to keep within a 2kg (4¼lb) range. And keep your food diary from time to time. Regular checks will keep you focused on the importance of keeping those new good habits firmly established.

Six Steps to Freedom

1   Stay real. Forget about fad diets and 'how to be skinny' pornography and propaganda.
2   Stay aware of the toxic environment and the power it, and your body's responses to it, can have.
3   Keep up some form of self-monitoring and ongoing support.
4   Practise conscious choice and 'flexible restraint'.
5   Don't panic if you go off track or gain a few pounds – you have the skills to survive and restabilize.
6   Enjoy being the one who is responsible and in charge – your self-belief will enhance other areas of your life, too.

How to Stay on Track – Secrets of the Successful

It's time for more inspiration from people who've been there, done that and stayed slimmer – for years.

The Lean Habits Study is currently under way in Germany and is investigating the weight and eating habits of nearly 7000 people over three years. After one year, those who were most successful at keeping their weight off after the 8–10 week weight-loss period tended to:

- Practise flexible restraint (see page 147).
- Have regular meals, at regular times and with little or no snacking.
- Improve the quality of their diet with more fruit and vegetables and other low-fat foods.
- Pay attention to their portion sizes.
- Sit down to eat their meals and take time over them, paying attention to what they were eating.
- Cope better with stress.

In Step One I described a study in the *American Journal of Clinical Nutrition*, and what strategies best helped women to lose weight. The study also looked at what they did to keep that weight off (or never become overweight in the first place). To remind you, the three groups of women questioned were:

- Maintainers (lost weight then stayed at their goal weight for at least two years).
- Relapsers (lost and regained their excess weight a number of times).
- Controls (always been a healthy weight).

Compared to 'relapsers', weight loss 'maintainers' tended to:

- Stay aware that they needed to be more active and conscious of the quantity and type of food they continued to eat – and carry this out.
- Regularly check their weight on the scales (but not obsessively). Some also used how their clothes fitted as a guide.
- Not tell themselves off if they overate, or feel guilty about eating certain foods.
- Be satisfied with their bodies.
- Have three regular meals and fewer snacks, especially confectionery.

How to unplug a weight control block (or a major lapse)

It happens to the best of us. You have been steadily losing weight, staying positive, making healthy choices and you feel close to your realistic goal weight. Or you have been maintaining your healthy weight for a few months now. But suddenly you just seem to 'lose it'. You want to eat with gay abandon. You rebel. You can't seem to stop. So what can you do?

- Forgive yourself – until you do that you simply can't get back on track.
- Write down all the reasons why weight control is important to you.
- Speak to people who are positive and manage their weight successfully.
- Take things day by day. Weight control is a long-term process with inevitable ups and downs, not something you only have one chance at. You haven't 'ruined everything'.
- If you weigh yourself and find your weight has gone up a few pounds remember that much of this is fluid, not fat, since you can't gain fat that quickly.
- Go back to keeping a thorough diary. Look out for negative self-talk and for 'head hunger' eating. Be honest, not critical. Use the diary to identify problem areas and plan ways to tackle them (see Step Four).
- Do a reality check – restart your food diary and find some time to have a think about what is going on in your life right now. Is it superstressful? Are you feeling angry about something? Do you have needs that aren't being met and food comes to the rescue?
- Deal with your reality check – plan what you can do, and what help you might need.
- Get back on track – after a few days of assessing the situation, get back to your meal plan. It is normal to go off track from time to time. Learn from your lapse. You know you can do it – you've been doing it for weeks, if not months..
- Get some support – from a helpful partner or friend, books, Internet communities, a slimming group or a health professional. Make sure they understand your current 'block'.
- Find something else to focus on. With all your new vitality there may be many things you can do now that you couldn't do before. For inspiration, look back at the things you felt your weight once stopped you doing.

- Manage stress and confront problems rather than eat, drink, sleep or wish they would go away.
- Use help and support from family, friends or professionals to help them deal with problems.

The women in the 'control' group reported similar strategies, and saw themselves not as women without a weight problem, but as women who consciously 'stayed in shape'. If they gained weight after a holiday they would lose it again when they returned home. One woman said: 'You won't be interested in me as I only eat when I am hungry, and then eat what I like, but in small quantities.'

The third study centres on the US National Weight Control Registry, which investigated the strategies of over 700 men and women who had been obese for some time, and had lost an average of 30kg (4stone 10lb) and kept it off for five years. They tended to:
- Eat breakfast.
- Continue to eat a low-fat diet.
- Not avoid any foods, but limit the amount of certain foods.
- Eat regular meals.
- Occasionally eat out, but limit fast food.
- Regularly monitor what they eat, e.g. with a food diary or in their head, counting calories or grams of fat.
- Regularly check their weight – once or twice a week.
- Continue to be more active – on average they exercised for an hour daily, for example, walked about 4 miles over the day.
- Lose weight more gradually than 'relapsers'.
- Manage not to fall into the trap of feeling guilty about eating too much, or a 'bad' food, and end up eating even more ('all or nothing' thinking).

Other points from this study
- Subjects who entered the study with higher levels of problems such as

depression, binge-eating and 'all or nothing' thinking about overeating were less likely to be successful for more than a year.

- The longer people had kept their weight off, the more likely they were to continue to succeed, no doubt because they had had time to practise new skills and attitudes, and allow their lifestyle changes to become permanent habits.

In summary, what these studies tell us is that ongoing attitude and lifestyle changes are fundamental to long-term weight control success. How we think and feel, determines what we do. The skills outlined throughout *Diet Trials* will help you to adopt new attitudes, goals and lifestyle choices, in preference to past unhelpful ones.

STRESS MANAGEMENT

Different things may stress different people, but stress is something we all experience. At the right level it can be something we benefit from. But if it gets too much it can be harmful to health and well-being, and is also a major trigger for overeating or making unhealthy food choices. Learning to recognize and manage stress, not feed it, is a key skill learnt by successful slimmers. In other words, those who manage stress do well at keeping their weight off long term.

Stress can come from different sources: from other people, work, events and life around us, and from unrealistic expectations or pressures that we put on ourselves. Some sources of stress can't be changed – for example, we can't stop a train running late – but we can change how we respond to them.

Stress is not just upsetting and anxiety-making; it unleashes a whole range of hormonal and chemical actions in the body. And if we don't counterbalance them in some way they can affect not just how and what we eat, but, over time, they can increase our risk of problems such as low resistance to infection, high blood pressure, migraine, bowel disorders, eczema, back pain and diabetes (stress hormones seem to make the body store more fat around the waist, see page 22).

When we are busy it is hard to find the time to relax properly, so we automatically look for stress relievers. Food can become a quick and effective 'stress fix' – and it soon becomes a learned response (see page 134). Some people may go off food when they are extremely stressed. But overeating in response to moderate stress is more common, and is a common cause of 'head hunger' eating (see page 136). Take some time to think about what stresses you have in your life at the moment, how they affect you and how you feel you respond to them. Write all this down if it helps.

If you feel that stress makes it harder for you to control and maintain your weight, think about how you could manage it better. Different approaches work for different people. Like all new skills it's a matter of practice and seeing what works best for you. These are some approaches that help with stress:

- Regular physical activity (see Step Five).
- Massage or 'release' of tension spots such as shoulders, neck, jaw and lower back. To release them, first clench or tighten and then relax them. Do this a couple of times.
- Breathing exercises – concentrating on regular deep breathing helps the body relax and tension ebb away. Breathe in, counting from one to four then breathe out counting from one to six or eight.
- Meditation, visualization and relaxation techniques.
- Learning to deal with the chain of negative thoughts, self-talk and consequential feelings and actions triggered by stress (see Step Four).
- Plan how to use your time efficiently, so that you don't feel as though you are constantly rushing from one thing to another. This is likely to mean saying 'No' to some things people ask you to do. Think of your needs as well as the needs of others.
- Use a food and thoughts diary to make a note of stressful events, and your responses to them.

Healthy Family Living

We all want the best for our families, and good health is no exception. Sometimes we take it for granted, or maybe we don't always know the best way to stay fit and healthy – or realize the impact our lifestyle has on our well-being.

Diet Trials has aimed to address this by providing motivating information about the basics of healthy living, together with practical skills that will help you to do what's important for you, and your family. Since healthy living can sometimes involve changing lifelong habits, be patient. Take things a step a time, don't be discouraged if things don't go as well as planned, and focus on what is most relevant to you. As you have read, realistic weight control is a vital part of our overall health and well-being – it's not just a cosmetic, or even a competitive, issue. It certainly isn't a feminist issue either – there are more overweight men than women, and serious concerns about rapidly rising weights amongst children.

There will always be a delicate balance to achieve between promoting healthy weight control and not causing anxiety about weight or shape. With children, there is the added concern of ensuring their diet isn't nutritionally restricted, to allow optimal growth and development. But the worldwide recognition of the epidemic of obesity, the toxic environment and the vast health problems they both bring, mean that messages about the importance of healthy and realistic weight control should become the desirable 'norm'. The key thing is to focus on why health rather than appearance is important; and on what is realistic – being a weight that is healthy and comfortably achieved, rather than 'fashionably' slim.

Meanwhile, be a good role model to your children. Think carefully about the way you might talk about weight and use food in family life – for comfort, love and to fill bored moments. Involve your children in food shopping and preparation where possible, and try to promote a

Surviving a Weight Loss Plateau

When you are losing weight it is very common to go through weeks when your weight stays much the same. This can be very discouraging but it can be overcome. You will need all your 'relapse prevention' skills (see page 146) to be in good working order if you are to stay positive.

First of all, make sure your weight-loss goal really is achievable. If it isn't, and you don't meet your expectations, you are likely to feel as though you've failed, and give up. Remember: most people find it hard to lose more than 10 per cent of their weight – at any one time.

If you decide your goal is realistic and have stopped keeping your food diary – make this a priority. A plateau is very often down to old habits, such as more 'head hunger' eating, less care about portion sizes and nibbling, creeping back in. Or you may be less active day to day, or might benefit from a bit more activity – walking a bit longer or building in some weight training. Note that if you are doing a lot more exercise you are likely to have gained more muscle. Although, on the scales, this may make it look as though you're not losing weight, you may still be losing body fat. (See page 23 for ways to better assess this.)

If you have plateau'd for a few weeks or so despite addressing the points above, and have already lost quite a bit of weight – say 10kg (1½ stone) or more – the plateau is probably because your calorie needs have gone down. This is not because you have ruined your metabolism, but because there is less of you to burn energy on a day-to-day basis. This means that to keep gradually losing weight, you will need to tip the balance in your favour by reducing your calorie intake or being more active, or ideally, a bit of both. A total calorie deficit of up to 250 to 300 calories a day should get things moving again.

Once you get to your realistic and healthier goal weight, remember that, for the reasons given above, the number of calories you will need to keep your weight stable will be lower than the number you needed before you lost weight.

This is another reason why it's so important to make lifestyle changes that you can keep to, rather than slipping back to old ways once a 'diet' is over.

sense of enjoyment of it as part of family life. After all, food and meal times are one of life's great pleasures.

See providing a healthy lifestyle as a positive and responsible part of caring for your children – not a negative way of depriving them, or yourself. Keep learning about how to survive the toxic environment, support those who are making lifestyle changes (and seek support for your changes) and build and preserve self-esteem through your family's many wonderfully unique abilities and achievements.

It's all worth it, especially since we only get one lifetime. Don't be too hard on yourself, either. You can't get everything 'just right'. Life, and being a parent, friend or partner, isn't that simple. But you can set realistic goals and keep giving them your best shot. The rewards will let you know that you've done your best.

section
3

weighing up popular ways

to lose weight

Have you ever tried a popular diet, club or pill? If so, what was your experience? Was it helpful, a disaster, short-lived, expensive, convenient? And how on earth did you choose what to go for?

Today, there are thousands of different books, pills, potions, clubs, magazines, special foods, supplements, gadgets, Internet sites, therapists, patches and clinics all offering ways to fight the flab. They have always been around but with the rise in overweight and obesity – and therefore the potential profits to be made – the range of choices is on the increase. The trouble is, as company profits get bigger so do our waistlines – suggesting these ways of losing weight don't really help. But is that fair? Are some products and programmes better than others? And if so, how can you wade through the information overload to find one that is safe and potentially effective?

In this section I will give a quick rundown of the most popular weight-loss approaches. You may think that because I have written this book and in it given 'fad' or 'quick-fix' diets a bit of a hard time, I am hardly likely to have much good to say about other ways of losing weight! But you might be surprised. Partly because different approaches suit different people, and partly because this book can nicely complement the responsible ones that suit you best. I say 'responsible' because I am not about to let fad or quick-fix diets off the hook! See page 195 for the British Dietetic Association's view on these.

The reason this book can go hand in hand with other approaches is because it provides sound information for building your skills and confidence in making long-term lifestyle changes; changes that are essential for success no matter what diet or medical treatment you follow initially. Responsible weight-loss clubs, Internet sites or health coaches can provide additional 'hands on' or interactive support while you are losing weight. And many have the scope to offer much more detailed information about meal planning or activity than there has been room for in this book. So, hopefully these resources will reinforce a lot of what's in *Diet Trials*. And, of course, you may already be receiving individualized advice from a doctor, dietitian or health professional at your doctor's surgery or privately.

The main reason this book is so fundamental to your success is that it helps you to take charge and believe in yourself. From the outset, it has encouraged you to ask yourself what is really important to you, not others, and then build your confidence in your abilities to control your weight. Knowledge, skills, realistic and sustainable goals, and clear motivations all contribute to that confidence, and allow you to take responsibility rather than relying on 'it' to make you lose weight. 'It' being the next diet, club, pill, or diet book – including this one! No matter how responsible and thorough a weight-loss approach is, 'it' can't make you lose weight. 'It' can only provide you with structure, information and support. The rest is up to you. The six steps of skills in *Diet Trials* will help you to make the most of whichever approach you decide suits you best.

Check out your attitude to diets

Before buying or signing up to a new weight-loss programme, ask yourself:
- Do I think 'it' will make me lose weight?
- Am I starting out thinking that I am quite an OK person right now, or do I think that can only happen once I lose the weight?
- Do I believe in my ability to take long-term responsibility for my weight and my health – or am I relying on 'it' to do it for me?

If you think the diet alone is your answer to weight loss and happiness, and you are serious about slimming success, I suggest you reread this book carefully before you embark on any weight loss programme.

And remember – it's important that you don't miss out the quizzes and questionnaires!

weighing up popular ways to lose weight   193

How to Assess Whether a Popular Diet or Weight-Loss Programme is Responsible or Not

To decide whether a book, club, programme or individual will provide the best support for you to develop the skills for long-term weight control, first find out how well it measures up to responsible ones. The more YES replies to these questions, the better:

▪ Is it written, developed or run by people with suitable qualifications and experience – for example, a state-registered dietitian, medical doctor, clinical psychologist, accredited fitness instructor?

▪ Is it based on scientifically sound advice?

▪ Does it *not* pretend to make weight loss effortless, or *not* suggest that you can 'eat as much, or as many calories as you like' and still lose weight?

▪ Is its overall aim to work towards long-term lifestyle and attitude changes – rather than a short-term, quick-fix approach?

▪ Does it incorporate the basic principles of balanced, healthy eating?

▪ Does it put the health benefits of weight loss before appearance?

▪ Does it help you to believe in your abilities and encourage you to feel OK about yourself whatever weight you are?

▪ Does it allow you to assess your weight and decide on realistic and healthy weight targets?

▪ Does it suggest a maximum weight loss of 0.45kg–0.9kg (1–2lb) a week, and emphasize that this is great progress?

▪ Does it recognize that people may not lose weight every week and, if they don't, does it offer them problem-solving support, rather than a telling off?

▪ Does it suggest who should seek medical or dietetic advice rather than follow the diet?

▪ Does it promote a positive attitude about food and help you to fit food into your life, rather than having lists of 'forbidden' foods?

- Does it aim to equip you with the skills and confidence to ultimately develop the flexible eating pattern that will best meet your needs? In other words, help you to find 'what works for you'?
- Does it recommend regular physical activity and provide practical and safe advice about how to be more active?
- Does it include simple behaviour change techniques – for example, keeping a food diary, identifying triggers, dealing with negative thoughts, coping with lapses?
- Does it advise against the use of slimming aids with unsubstantiated claims – for example, those offering painless, rapid weight loss, 'fat burners' or high-dose supplements?
- Does it provide or recommend some form of ongoing support – for example, from a group, friend, family member or health professional?

The British Dietetic Association has the following advice on how to spot fad or quick-fix diets.

It's a 'quick-fix' or fad diet if it...
- Recommends strange quantities of only one or a few foods – for example, grapefruit, meat, eggs, or soup.
- Promotes 'magical' foods to 'burn' fat. You only lose weight when you eat fewer calories than your body needs and/or are more active. No foods actually burn fat.
- Suggests rigid menus, greatly limiting food choice, and the times of day you can eat.
- Advises that foods should only be eaten in specific combinations.
- Suggests rapid weight loss of more than 2lbs (1kg) a week.
- Doesn't address barriers to changing eating habits.
- Fails to recommend regular physical activity.
- Doesn't warn people with diabetes, high blood pressure, a kidney disorder or other medical conditions to seek medical advice before starting the diet.

POPULAR WAYS OF LOSING WEIGHT UNCOVERED

Now for a quick tour around the most popular ways people choose to lose weight. I will give a quick outline of what each involves, whether there is any evidence to support how effective it is and any obvious pros and cons. Then it's up to you to decide; I am not here to say what you should or shouldn't do. Just to make sure you are aware of what lies behind the sometimes 'interesting' claims. And don't forget the all-important issue of staying well nourished while you are losing weight. This is important for everyone, and particularly for women who may be planning to have a baby.

At the end of the day, if you find an approach to weight control that helps you to feel good about yourself, lets you stay at a healthier weight, is nutritionally sound and doesn't stop you enjoying life, you can't ask for much more than that. Don't forget to use the guidance on page 195 to help you reach a verdict.

Meal Replacements

What are they?

Meal replacements are designed to replace two meals and so enable you to consume fewer calories than you burn, and lose weight. The products are said to give people a simple and structured, calorie-controlled eating pattern, making using them easier than following diets with a wider choice of food.

Examples of products in the UK are Slim.Fast, Boots Shapers and Tesco's Ultra Slim. Typically, you might replace breakfast and lunch with a meal replacement product, such as a shake, soup or pasta dish and have a balanced meal – providing around 600 calories – in the evening. Two to three low-fat snacks such as fruit, low-fat soups or a snack bar are also advised to ensure a total of 1200 to 1400 calories over the day. Users are advised to drink at least six to eight glasses of water or other low-calorie liquids daily. The products are fortified with vitamins and minerals and provide protein, carbohydrate, fat and fibre. Their nutritional composition and labelling is controlled by EU legislation.

Some products come with printed and Internet guides to healthy living, and include information about healthy eating, being more active and changing eating habits. So if you decide to try them, make sure you use this information. Once weight is lost, the usual advice is to use one meal replacement a day alongside new healthy habits to help keep the weight off.

Are they useful and responsible?

Published studies show that proper use of meal replacements can provide a nutritionally balanced diet. The replacements have also enabled people who stay with the programme (a certain proportion of subjects always drops out of studies), to lose an average of 10 per cent of their weight, and keep it off in study periods ranging from one to four years. But these were subjects in a research study who had extra face-to-face support and education. They were not people who simply buy the products from the shelves – as most ordinary consumers would do – and therefore don't have the same help and support in developing the skills to change their eating and activity habits once they stop using the products. At the moment, we don't know how useful meal replacements are when they are used in this way. But the approach appears to be safe and effective, and meets most of the assessment criteria. These products could be used to help achieve the recommended modest 5 to 10 per cent weight loss if the meal plans are followed, especially if people enlist some form of ongoing support (see page 213). While weight-loss plans using meal replacements may not suit everyone, they are one option.

Slimming Clubs

What are they?

Slimming clubs are, typically, weekly fee-paying events. They have their own eating plans, and recommend regular physical activity as well as giving advice on lifestyle changes. Setting goal weights and a weekly 'weigh-in' are also typical. The best-known commercial slimming clubs in the UK include Rosemary Conley Diet & Fitness Clubs, Weight Watchers and Slimming World. A meeting may consist of a weigh-in followed by a lecture on a particular subject, and a group discussion. Some clubs may have exercise classes. Each will have its own rules about fees and attendance. Weight maintenance programmes may be offered.

Are they useful and responsible?

There is very limited published research about the long-term effectiveness of slimming clubs, which is a pity, and hopefully more will come. But what there is suggests that responsible clubs could be useful. One study suggests they may be more useful than self-help programmes but it was only carried out over a six-month period. Before joining any club I would encourage you to find out what it offers and ask yourself what you see as its benefits for you. Most importantly, see if it offers some form of ongoing support to help you maintain your weight loss. The well-known clubs in the UK generally meet the assessment criteria, but small, independent clubs should be looked at more carefully.

Clubs can offer important group support and encouragement that you don't get from most other methods. Remember, though, despite often detailed or novel diet plans, lectures, information booklets and exercise programmes, clubs still can't make you lose weight – you have to feel ready and able to go into action, on your own terms. So don't feel intimidated by any pressure to lose a certain amount of weight each week. And question any tactics that make you feel 'naughty' rather than 'supported' if you don't lose – and indeed gain. And if you feel you would benefit from more individualized advice, clubs may not be for you. Some, however, also offer Internet and home-based programmes. Overall responsible clubs offer good-quality information, keep up to date with current health advice, help with problem solving and offer maintenance programmes, and so could help you make the necessary lifestyle changes to achieve modest weight loss and long-term weight control.

Internet Sites

What are they?

There is a growing number of Internet sites offering slimming solutions. These can vary greatly in quality and range from supplement sales to comprehensive weight-loss programmes with individualized support via e-mail. Most offer some level of free information, but a fee is required for more individualized advice and information. The more comprehensive sites, for example, www.realslimmers.com and www.edietsuk.co.uk, generally offer chat-room communities, recipes, features to help build skills relating to diet, exercise and behaviour change, health assessment tools and news updates. Many, for example, www.tntgetfit.com and www.cyberdiet.com, also offer meal plans which are said to be designed to meet your needs. Some sites, such as www.fatmanslim.com, provide ongoing support for people once they've lost weight, using a home-based weight-control package.

Are they useful and responsible?

There is limited published information about Internet sites, but one American study did find that after six months, and after an initial face-to-face consultation, people using a responsible site lost an average of

1.7kg (3¾lb). This increased to 4.1kg (9lb) if they received weekly lessons in how to change behaviour, and kept food records.

A recent report into Internet slimming by the consumer magazine *Health Which?* concluded that only one out of 10 comprehensive sites reviewed had relatively good practice when giving individualized advice. They recommend that you look for sites that use state-registered dietitians (or registered dietitians for US sites) and other qualified health professionals – as well as checking them against the points outlined in the assessment criteria on page 195. Sites that carry 'Health on the Net' symbols have been assessed by external bodies, but it's still worth making up your mind for yourself.

Again, different approaches suit different people and if your lifestyle means clubs are out of the question, and you have easy access to the Internet, the convenience of this approach may suit you. The chat rooms offer 'instantly accessible' support too. But you do have to be self-motivated to use them properly – and will need to keep the contact up or find other ways to help you with weight maintenance. Choose carefully, and remember, 'it' can't do it for you.

Diet or Health Coaches

What are they?

A health coach will ask you about your eating habits as a way of helping you to get to the source of any problems. Rather than giving advice, coaches challenge you to be honest with yourself and take responsibility for your own health and eating patterns. They have a starting point that overeating is not about food but simply a symptom of a deeper issue. For example, are you using food to comfort yourself, to suppress your feelings or to alleviate boredom? A coach will ask you to design your own healthy eating plan, because the theory is that you know what's best for you. Some health coaches will coach by telephone; others will see you face-to-face and may use hypnotherapy or neurolinguistic programming (NLP) as part of the coaching. In many ways coaching 'techniques' are similar to cognitive behavioural therapy and motivational interviewing approaches – many of which are outlined in this book.

Are they useful and responsible?

Coaching is still a fairly new profession. To check out your coach's professional qualifications go to the website for the governing body – The International Coach Federation at www.coachfederation.org.

There is little published work on the effectiveness of coaching, but there is some evidence that it can help dietary change over a six-month period. Like this book, it draws strongly and positively on the belief that how you think affects how you feel and how you act. A health coach may not necessarily have sound knowledge about nutrition or physical activity, so be aware of this. As usual, use the assessment guide, and talk to the coach about what is involved, including the cost. If you feel it's right for you, it may well help you to achieve modest weight-loss goals.

Diet Books – in General

When it comes to diet books there's certainly something for everyone – low or high carbohydrate, low or high fat, sexy, X-rated, cabbagey or blood-group-based – you name it. It does make you wonder how each can work in its own unique way, and how some can claim to hold the latest scientific breakthrough in diet, health and weight loss!

Some diet books pull no punches. They make it clear that their approach is to help you cut calories, and set about giving rules, regulations and practical suggestions on how to do just that. While the quality of the advice can vary greatly, they are not trying to offer a new 'theory' on weight loss.

Popular diet books with eating rules that lead to large weight losses in the short term – thanks to their low calorie level and its effects on both fluid and fat loss (see page 33) – are understandably very appealing, but there is currently scant evidence that they help in the long term. There is also no published scientific evidence to support any claims that weight loss is due to any reason other than consuming fewer calories than you burn. I am not saying that I have all the answers either. No one has. And sometimes people who are very obese, and have not been successful with more conventional approaches, find that a more novel and medically monitored approach to the weight-loss phase of weight control helps them most. Published papers on the long-term outcome – the all-important weight-maintenance phase of weight control – of any weight-loss method are limited. But the evidence is strongest for behaviour changes based on healthy, balanced eating, combined with increased physical activity and a positive and flexible way of thinking about food, weight and day-to-day life (see page 34).

So, before being lured by the promise of effortless weight loss or celebrity testimonials, see how your chosen diet measures up to the assessment criteria. You may well find it lacking. Especially in the area of developing the skills to set and achieve realistic and sustainable goals. Some of the food recommendations may be interesting, too – and limited food choice can mean that diets don't provide enough essential vitamins and minerals, or are difficult to make part of your work or social and family life. And physical activity sometimes doesn't even get a look in.

But most importantly, could the book help you to believe in your own abilities, feel good about yourself, and make the necessary lifestyle and attitude changes that successful slimmers swear by?

Low-Carbohydrate Diets

What are they?

These diets involve basing meals on meat, poultry, fish, eggs, cheese and salad vegetables. They severely restrict all carbohydrate-rich foods such as bread, potatoes, pasta, pizza, chocolate, crisps, cereals and sugars and limit most fruits, some vegetables and many alcoholic drinks. Liberal use of butter, oil and fatty meats is permitted in some versions. While more carbohydrate is permitted in weight-maintenance phases of the diets, the overall dietary recommendations are still quite different from the international and evidence-based consensus for both good health and weight control.

Are they useful and responsible?

The American Heart Association, along with many other health professional groups, does not recommend them for the general public. Neither do I. There is published evidence to show that people do lose weight on low-carbohydrate diets, but in most cases weight loss and calorie restriction by any means will improve things like high blood fats, blood glucose and blood pressure. However, despite claims that weight loss is due to the low carbohydrate intake and the effect this has on lowering levels of insulin in the blood rather than eating fewer calories, scientific reviews have found no evidence to substantiate this.

While these diets may suit some people there is no special magic to them; they're just low-calorie diets with a novel set of dietary rules and restricted food choice. This means that you eat fewer calories than usual, and lose weight. Vitamin and mineral supplements are needed as the diets are not nutritionally adequate. We also don't know how they might affect our health if followed long term – studies suggest that they may increase the risk of kidney stones and cause the body to lose more potassium and calcium. They are not suitable for people with medical conditions such as kidney disease or gout or for pregnant women.

Cutting back on sugary and refined carbohydrate-rich foods is a good idea, but you don't need to go to such extremes. A main concern about widespread public use of these diets is that they restrict health-protecting carbohydrate-rich foods such as whole grains and many fruits and vegetables. And unless lean meats and low-fat cheeses are chosen, intake of saturated fat is high. The diets are also difficult to cope with socially, can be expensive, cause constipation and offer little support for behaviour changes and 'getting your head straight' (see page 131). As with many popular diets and programmes there is also currently no evidence that 'low carb' diets help people control their weight in the long term, which after all is what it's about.

Food-Combining Diets

What are they?

Food-combining diets claim that certain foods should not be combined at the same meal because this interferes with proper digestion. Books about these diets usually suggest that calories don't count when it comes to weight loss, and that food combining can restore weight to its natural levels.

Dietary rules vary from book to book, but the basics are that protein-rich foods such as meat, fish, eggs and dairy products should not be eaten at the same meal as carbohydrate-rich foods (bread, cereals, potatoes, rice, pasta, noodles and sugary foods). Other vegetables, salad and most fruit can be eaten with either a protein-rich or carbohydrate-rich meal. Between-meal snacks of 'neutral' foods are usually permitted. Any form of processed food is discouraged, so most meals are made from 'natural' foods and require preparation.

Are they useful and responsible?

If you follow one of these diets and lose weight it's because the food rules mean you eat fewer calories than you burn – not because of food-combining principles, which are essentially nutritional nonsense. This has been proved in a controlled clinical trial when subjects ate either a food-combining diet or a standard, balanced weight-loss diet, both with the same calorie level, over a six-week period – and both groups lost the same amount of weight.

The fact that the diet restricts combinations of foods, stops people eating high-fat and sugary processed foods, and encourages them to eat more fruit and vegetables, is likely to lead to lower calorie intake – and potentially modest weight loss. Some books restrict red meat and dairy foods, so it's necessary to make wise choices to keep the diet balanced. A food-combining diet can be tricky when you are eating out, and there is a lot of cooking from scratch, which may not always suit busy people. If you can keep this approach up long term it could be healthy enough and help to keep the weight off. But books about these diets typically provide limited information on physical activity, 'getting your head straight' and behaviour changes to enhance that process.

Detox Diets

What are they?

Detox diets are based on the belief that our bodies are continually assaulted by an overload of 'toxins' such as pesticides, food additives, high-fat foods, pollution, drugs, caffeine, and alcohol. Detox is short for 'detoxification' – the process by which the body transforms these so-called toxins into substances that can be passed from the body. Most of these diets also claim that they can help you to lose weight.

Detox diets can vary greatly in content and length, but typically involve eating lots of organic fruit, vegetables, juices, herbal teas, nuts, seeds and brown rice, and drinking plenty of water, preferably bottled. They could last for two days to a week, or longer for less restrictive plans. Supplements may also be recommended. Foods that are usually banned are sugar, meat, wheat, dairy foods, salt, additives, canned and packaged foods, caffeine and alcohol.

Are they useful and responsible?

I am not aware of any published studies that directly compare detox and standard diets, but detox ones are likely to cause weight loss because the dietary restrictions mean you eat fewer calories than you usually do. No magic 'metabolism boosting' or 'cleansing' – just fewer calories. In terms of 'detox', we are actually designed with sophisticated systems to break down and excrete wastes, and while it makes sense to not overdo caffeine, alcohol, high-fat foods and exposure to pollutants, we can help our bodies withstand environmental toxins with a healthy, balanced diet, rather than with potentially restrictive regimens.

The diets are usually quite stringent, food must be self-prepared and some ingredients might be hard to find or expensive, not to mention novel to taste buds. Whole food groups are sometimes omitted, especially the calcium-rich milk and dairy group, so it's vital to ensure that nutritious alternatives are found to keep your diet nutritionally adequate. The high fibre content can make for embarrassing wind, and sudden caffeine withdrawal (and a low food intake) can cause headaches. The short-term and rigid nature of detox diets, and the lack of behaviour-change support, puts them into the 'quick-fix' category – and makes them low scorers on the assessment criteria. But, they might be helpful if they are viewed as a way to kick-start healthier habits – for example, eating more fruit and vegetables and less fatty and sugary foods. However, there are ways of achieving this, and long-term weight control success, that are far less extreme but nutritionally balanced.

Low Glycaemic Index (GI) Diets

What are they?

The glycaemic index (GI) is the ranking of foods according to how quickly they cause a rise in blood glucose levels (see page 87). Research suggests that diets rich in foods with a low GI help you to feel fuller for longer, and so help you to control your weight. They also seem to have beneficial effects on blood glucose and blood fat levels, as well insulin levels. A number of popular diet books use the GI as part of their recommendations – some more accurately than others. So look for books written by qualified and reputable health and medical professionals.

Are they useful and responsible?

Low-GI diets will help you to lose weight as long as they provide diet and exercise information that allows you to eat fewer calories than you burn. There are currently few studies that look specifically at the weight-control effects of low-GI diets, but the more reputable books promote diet plans that are basically fine-tuned versions of standard healthy eating advice. On page 88, I recommend making low-GI foods part of meals and snacks whenever possible. Using the principles of low-GI eating within a calorie-controlled eating plan will promote modest weight loss, but this will only be sustained with long-term changes. Most books about these diets give practical guidance and promote physical activity, but may be lacking when it comes to support for making sustained lifestyle changes and 'getting your head straight'. Make sure the meal plans are practical and nutritionally balanced.

Supplements

What are they?

The supplements referred to here are ones that contain various ingredients that do things like 'burn fat', 'let you lose weight while you sleep', 'boost metabolism', 'absorb fat', 'suppress appetite', 'build muscle and lose fat' and 'fill you up'. Most come with calorie-controlled diet plans. Some of the claims are obviously ridiculous (but still tempting!) while others have something to them. The hard part is knowing which supplement might help and which one is just a waste of your money.

Are they useful and responsible?

Any supplement making a claim that it can promote weight loss by any means other than helping you to consume fewer calories must provide published scientific evidence to support that view. Even then, if it is truly effective it should have to go through the rigorous controls that medicines go through, because it must be doing something that affects how the body functions – for example, by significantly stimulating the metabolic rate. And because supplements aren't tested like medicines, there is rarely information on how safe it is to take them for long periods.

The bottom line is that most supplements cannot live up to their claims and have no real benefits for long-term weight control. The most useful part is probably the low-calorie diet plan that comes with them, plus your enthusiasm to lose weight after spending so much money – for a while anyway! And the claims for many are cleverly worded to entice you but not break trading standards laws. Some weight-loss supplements sold by mail order by companies based abroad are total scams. So, if it sounds too good to be true, it probably is! Supplements that studies have shown to be effective in helping you to feel fuller for longer show the most promise – but they still work by helping you to eat fewer calories than you burn (which they make clear), so they are not magic bullets.

Before taking the plunge and buying a supplement, ask yourself:
1   Does it include a guide to who the product is not suitable for, or who should consult a doctor before trying to lose weight?
2   Does it help you to assess your current weight, and recommend healthy rates of weight loss?
3   Does it claim to effect weight loss for reasons other than helping you to eat fewer calories than you burn?
4   Does it provide information about published clinical trials to support any claims it makes?

Segmented Plates and Traffic-Light Guides

What are they?

There are many gadgets and aids that can help you change how much and what you eat. One example is a segmented plate, which allows you to serve yourself healthy proportions of foods for your main meals, in line with the 'Balance of Good Health' (see page 67). It guides you towards half-filling your plate with vegetables or salad and having smaller proportions of carbohydrate- and protein-rich foods. Another guide can help you to classify proportions of foods according to a traffic-light system (green = go for it; amber = caution; red = danger) and comes complete with guidance on portion sizes to keep your diet calorie controlled and balanced.

Are they useful and responsible?

These tools have not been tested for effectiveness in formal studies, but are based on sound nutritional principles and may be helpful for skill-building around food. However, they aren't weight-control programmes in themselves.

MEDICAL APPROACHES TO WEIGHT CONTROL

Doctors and the health professionals who work with them – the primary care team – are interested in what their patients weigh. In the past, they may not always have got too involved. But times have changed, thanks to the chilling evidence about the effects that obesity has on our health. When you think about it, obesity could be described as one of our greatest 'silent' killers. Illnesses linked to it could shave nine years off potential lifespans and cause much ill health and poor quality of life. And, as well as that tremendous personal cost, there is the cost to the NHS and UK economy, estimated to be at least £2.5 billion a year.

Health professionals know that the needs of many overweight and obese people have long been overlooked, and want to address that. Groups such as the National Obesity Forum, Dietitians Working in Obesity Management (UK) and the Association for the Study of Obesity (see page 200) are working to raise the profile of obesity treatment, improve services for patients and develop standards of care. More doctors, nurses and dietitians are working to improve their skills to provide treatment for patients. But you will still find that some doctors and health professionals are more interested than others in obesity treatment and sometimes you may need to raise the issue yourself.

But no matter how good intentions are, because over half of all adults are overweight, and one in five is obese, health-care resources simply can't stretch to provide help for everyone. Not that everyone wants help from his or her doctor, of course. Many people will manage very well by themselves, or with the help of responsible books or clubs. But others, despite their best efforts, need more assistance – especially if they have been obese for a long time, have an associated medical condition or are very obese (a BMI of 35 or more). Remember, many factors, including our genetic make-up, impact on our weight, and for some these influences are too strong to manage without additional help. That's why obesity is viewed as a complex medical condition.

When you see your doctor about your weight, he or she will assess it using the different methods described in Section One. They should also assess: any other medical problems (they are likely to take blood tests); your lifestyle; your readiness to make the changes required to lose weight and any potential barriers; your past 'dieting' experiences; and your current eating and activity habits. As you know, a wide range of health problems are linked to obesity – diabetes, high blood pressure, breathlessness or back pain, for example – and reaching a healthier weight can be a vital part of treating them (see page 13).

Your doctor can talk this through with you and make recommendations, but unless you feel ready to make changes no one can force you. Perhaps unsurprisingly, one of the most common motivators for people (especially men) to lose weight, is bad health news from their doctor. It certainly gives you something to think about. And if you really do feel that you want to lose weight for your health's sake, but feel that you can't do it alone, there are a number of options available. Your doctor will refer you on for the most appropriate support.

What Could Your Doctor Offer You?

Depending on the services that are available locally, and most importantly, what you feel will help you most, your doctor might suggest any of these possible options:

- Referral to an exercise prescription scheme at a local sports centre.
- Contact with local weight-control groups. These might be run by health professionals or be responsible slimming clubs.
- Referral to the practice nurse for weight-control advice based on

lifestyle changes and for ongoing support.

- Referral to a dietitian for further assessment and more specialist weight-control advice and ongoing support.
- Referral to a clinical psychologist for behavioural therapy.
- Referral to a counsellor, hypnotherapist or acupuncturist.
- Anti-obesity medication – to be used in conjunction with support from a health professional.
- Referral to a hospital obesity clinic. Doctors, dietitians, nurses, clinical psychologists, physiotherapists and surgeons with specialist skills are likely to be part of the hospital health-care team.

Medication or surgery is usually only recommended after lifestyle changes have been attempted for three to six months, but without success. The measure of 'success' is losing 5 to 10 per cent of weight in three months, together with improvement in known health problems – both physical and psychological. However, for some, weight maintenance, or any weight loss, is an important achievement and has positive effects on overall well-being.

Different Dietary Treatments That May be Offered for Weight Loss

Your doctor will probably refer you to the practice nurse, a dietitian who comes to the surgery or the dietitian at the local hospital, for dietary advice. State-registered dietitians are involved in training members of the primary care team. In Britain, there is only one NHS dietitian per 18,000 people!

The nurse or dietitian is likely to offer help with 'behaviour change' – which is similar to what's outlined in this book. Obviously, the length of appointments and their frequency are limited, but these health professionals will work with you, to help you to build the skills to set realistic goals and make lifestyle changes. You could potentially choose from either a 'goal-setting' approach, or a more structured 'food exchange' approach calculated to help you cut 600 calories from your current calorie needs. Sound familiar?

If you have tried lifestyle approaches, but have still been unable to lose, or keep off, enough weight to benefit your health problems, a dietitian, in conjunction with your doctor, may offer other dietary approaches. These may provide more thorough cognitive behavioural therapy support (see page 54) or they may combine this with a more novel dietary approach. Your doctor may refer you to a private weight-control programme if they are available locally.

When your health dictates the need for weight loss, novel diets are like medical treatments. They are usually followed for 12 to 16 weeks, which enables people to lose at least that beneficial 10 per cent of their weight. Regular support and help with building skills for weight maintenance using balanced dietary approaches is also provided. If people are extremely obese, the weight-loss period can be repeated again at a future date. Some of these dietary approaches may carry mild side effects or aren't suitable if people have certain medical conditions – which is why medical and dietetic guidance is so vital.

Dietary options as part of overall behaviour change and medical treatment could include:

- Meal replacements as part of a structured meal plan (see page 197).
- Very low-calorie diets (VLCDs). These are structured diets in which all meals are replaced by specific drinks, soups, bars or desserts which have been specially formulated and are nutritionally adequate – but typically provide 800 calories (some provide 500 calories). Salads, vegetables and fruit may be part of the plan, plus additional fluids.
- Milk diets. These are 800-calorie meal plans based on skimmed or semi-skimmed milk, with vitamin and mineral supplements, plus additional fluids.
- Modified carbohydrate diets.

Anti-Obesity Drugs

There are currently two drugs approved for use as part of the medical treatment of obesity. They have been developed in recognition of the fact that it is a complex disorder where, say, genetic effects on appetite are very difficult to manage, especially in the toxic environment. What they are not however, is a magic weight-loss bullet. The drugs must still be used as part of overall lifestyle changes – they just make that change more manageable for some people.

Both drugs come with strict criteria about who they can be prescribed for, and for how long. They are not for everyone, and they don't help everyone who is prescribed them. Orlistat works by reducing the amount of fat you absorb by about one-third, and must be taken with a low-fat diet (otherwise unpleasant bowel problems can result). Sibutramine helps you to feel more satisfied with less food by regulating the action of appetite-influencing chemical messengers in the brain (see page 28). Both work by reducing overall calorie intake – they don't 'melt fat' or send the metabolism into overdrive. And the clinical trials found that they don't make the stones drop off. Like other responsible treatments, they help people lose modest but beneficial amounts of weight.

These drugs have a recognized role to play in obesity treatment, and are very different from other drugs that might be available from private 'diet clinics' or even over the Internet. These include appetite suppressants and diuretics (which force the body to lose fluid). They are not recommended by the Royal College of Physicians. Avoid them.

You will no doubt read about 'new drug breakthroughs' and 'promising slimming pill research'. Because obesity is such a serious health problem, and because very obese people do find it difficult to control their weight, the hunt for new drugs is intense. Very often the reports are based on animal studies, or are the result of identifying one of the many genes or hormones that can influence weight. It is likely to be some time before new, effective drugs come on to the market, but they will no doubt arrive. Even then, there will be no getting away from the fact that skills to cope with the toxic environment will be fundamental to successful treatment. Medication can only aid weight control – long-term lifestyle changes and realistic goals remain the key.

Anti-Obesity Surgery

When extreme (or 'morbid') obesity becomes life-threatening and all other treatments have been tried, surgery to reduce stomach size is a final option. Bariatric surgery (as it is known) is currently not that common in the UK, but with the rise in the numbers of people who may benefit from it and the development of new procedures, it will no doubt become more widely available. Research indicates that for many people suffering from extreme obesity it can be a successful and life-changing option. People who want this surgery, and meet the medical criteria, have both their physical health and emotional well-being carefully assessed before any decisions are made. They are also fully informed of the potential benefits (and risks) of the procedures.

The most common procedure uses a gastric band that makes the stomach smaller, and so limits the amount that can be eaten at any one time. This is usually carried out as keyhole surgery, and the band can be surgically adjusted (to make the stomach smaller or larger) or removed if need be. Another procedure is the 'gastric bypass' which involves greatly reducing the size of the stomach as well as 'bypassing' some of the small intestine. This is a more complex operation and reduces both the amount of food that can eaten and the amount that is absorbed. This is an effective, but basically permanent, operation so it's vital to be aware that eating habits will change dramatically, and literally, for life. Specialized dietary advice as part of the medical follow-up is required after both these procedures, to help people adjust to their new small stomach, and keep their diet nutritionally adequate.

CASE STUDIES

Other people's weight-loss successes are always inspiring and can be very helpful to people who are just embarking on a weight-loss programme of their own. Here is a selection of real-life stories from successful slimmers that I hope will be an inspiration to you.

Graham, 44, has lost 4½ stone over the past year

'Being more aware of what's in food and knowing how to balance my overall calorie intake really helped, for example by "saving up" calories for a good night out or holiday, and using calorie-counted ready meals. Cutting down on the beer I was drinking helped too, especially since it was about habit rather than pleasure. I now feel much fitter and am back wearing favourite clothes. And it wasn't as difficult as I thought it would be, as I made my own choices and wasn't following a rigid diet!'

Liz, 30, (Graham's fiancée) has lost 2 stone over the past year

'Being able to share my daily thoughts and get support from Graham was great, as were food diaries, especially if I was having a rough patch. I also learned to feel more in control around food – very important since I work with it!

Making sure I still had some "treats" and being more choosy about what I ate rather than feel deprived was all part of that. And I stopped telling myself off if I did over-indulge, and just got back to it the next day. Doing more exercise was also vital as it helps me feel positive and manage stress better.'

William, 54, thought he couldn't lose weight but has lost 2 stone and kept it off

'I suddenly realized it was nonsense or excuses. The simple truth is that if you eat too many calories you gain weight. I stopped telling everyone that I ate little, drank no more beer than my slimmer friends, so it must be in my genes. I kept a food diary for a while and saw there was lots of bits creeping in. So I filled up on lower calorie foods, went for maximum satisfaction from anything I ate, learned to read labels and never said I was "on a diet" or "not allowed anything". And I could not have imagined all the benefits – feeling fitter, better sex life, comments from admiring women, no snoring and a much better back – it's really great.'

Nikky, 40, lost weight and gave up smoking

'I had tried to stop smoking once before, and gained 19kg (3 stone). But this time I approached it differently. I used nicotine replacement products for the first few months, then weaned myself off them, staying conscious of what I was eating, and why. I did gain about 3kg (half a stone), but I was prepared for that. I am now nicotine-free, my weight has stabilized, my asthma's a lot better and I'm confident that I'll get back to my healthier weight.'

Cirian, 28, regular exercise and 'trading off' helped her to lose 2 stone

'I had tried to lose weight every possible way since I was 14. I knew I should eat better and be more active, but it just felt too hard, or I was different in some way. Then I had a health scare. Before I knew the results it struck me that if they were positive I could do nothing about it. But I could control my weight. I finally realized that I had to take responsibility, and yes, it would be hard work. No more excuses, I had to confront reality. I then got into exercise – and am now a qualified fitness instructor! It's doubly amazing because I never did sport at school as I always felt too slow and embarrassed. By being so active I can eat more, and I consciously trade off, say exercise for a night out, or wine for chips! The exercise geared me mentally and physically towards being not just being a successful loser, but a weight loss maintainer. I will always stay active now, because it is part of my life.'

Anne, 38, lost 6 stone with the help of an interactive dietitian-led Internet site

'I am a very determined person, but didn't want everyone to know that I was losing weight. I also had a young baby, so the flexibility of the Internet was ideal. The meal plans and recipes from the site were useful, as it was not a rigid diet. If I get a craving, or am eating out, I will have a bit of what I fancy, otherwise I know I will just eat it eventually – on top of whatever else I've just eaten. That way I feel satisfied and end up eating less overall. I am much more aware of portion sizes of food I buy to eat at home too. We now do a lot of active things as a family, which is great exercise for me and for everyone.'

Pauline, 47, lost weight in her early 20s and has kept it off

'I first became "podgy" as a teenager. I wasn't obsessive about it, but felt that I could certainly eat more healthily, so just cut back in the stodge and upped the fruit and vegetables. And I have kept it off for all those years, even after having a baby. I enjoy food, but do keep a check on what I eat, and my weight. Friends who struggle with their weight think I am lucky because I stay slim. But it doesn't just happen. I feel that I can control my weight, not feel food controls me. And I don't think about food all the time – like my "struggling" friends. So yes I suppose I am lucky, but with a positive attitude others could be too.'

Peter, 59, lost 2 stone with a medically supervised, structured programme

'I now think totally differently about food. I am more active every day – I walk whenever I have the opportunity – as I know that means I can enjoy that extra glass of wine, or whatever. My mind set is now right, for life. I haven't been on a short-term diet, this is about long term change.

I have replaced old unhelpful habits with new, enjoyable ones, I never feel deprived, I continue to eat out a lot, my bad knee is better, and I feel much more positive overall.'

Diane, 27, slimming club stopped her quick-fix diets – and she has kept off 2 stone

'By the time I left University I was into crash dieting. The "soup diet", "fruit diet" and detox diets are the most memorable, or just skipping meals. But they made me feel hungry, tired and irritable. I always regained the weight too.

I realize now that I knew nothing about healthy eating, and even though I went to the gym I just thought it meant I could eat more. Holiday snaps finally made me join a responsible slimming group. The information and support I got made all the difference, and I felt really well. I now have a totally different attitude to food. I would never try another "guilt" diet because they make you feel awful, and they don't work.'

Greg, 28, 'walking is great'

'To be more active I usually feel I have to do some type of sport. But I don't always have time to be so organized. I recently started walking with a friend, and it's great. You see all sorts of things you don't see when you are driving, and it gives me time to think and talk about problems at work that are hard to reflect on when you're rushing around.'

Pete, 30, shift work and weight

'Changing to shift work really upset my diet, the weight started to go on, and I had real digestion problems. I went to see a dietitian for some advice. Apparently night shifts work against your body's circadian rhythms. They also meant it was easy to eat more junk food, and sugary drinks, partly to stay awake! I had to start planning ahead to make sure I took better food and drinks in with me. I was advised to have my main meal after getting up in the afternoon. Then at work to have healthy snacks every few hours.

Cutting right back on the caffeine and fizzy drinks eased my indigestion too – and helps me sleep better.'

USEFUL ORGANIZATIONS, FURTHER READING AND REFERENCES

Professional and academic associations and health charities

- Association for the Study of Obesity www.aso.org
- British Dietetic Association, tel 0121 200 8080, www.bda.uk.com
- British Heart Foundation, tel 0207 935 0185, www.bhf.org
- BHF Centre of Physical Activity and Health www.bhfactive.org.uk
- Diabetes UK, tel 0207 424 1000, www.diabetes.org.uk
- National Obesity Forum, tel 0115 8462109, www.nationalobesityforum.org.uk
- Weight Concern, tel 0207 679 6636, www.weightconcern.com
- USDA Center for Nutrition Policy and Promotion www.usda.gov/cnpp, www.nutrition.gov

Government agencies

- Department of Health, Social Services and Public Safety (Northern Ireland), tel www.dhsspsni.gov.uk
- Food Standards Agency www.foodstandards.gov.uk
- Health Education Board of Scotland, tel 0131 536 5500, www.hebs.scot.nhs.uk
- Health Promotion Wales www.hpw.wales.gov.uk

Further reading and websites

- *Fighting Fat, Fighting Fit*: BBC Worldwide Limited, 1999.
- *Ainsley Harriott's Low-Fat Meals in Minutes*: BBC Worldwide Limited, 2002
- *Good Food: 101 Low-Fat Faves*: BBC Worldwide Limited, 2003
- www.bbc.co.uk/diettrials
- www.bbc.co.uk/health

References

- Anderson J et al., Long term weight loss maintenance: a meta-analysis of US studies, *American Journal of Clinical Nutrition* 2001; 74(5): 579–84.
- Ashton D, *Healthy Heart Handbook for Women*, London:Vermilion, 2000.
- British Dietetic Association. Manual of Dietetic Practice. Oxford: Blackwell Science, 2001.
- British Nutrition Foundation, *Obesity*, Oxford: Blackwell Science, 1999.
- Astrup A, Dietary approaches to reducing body weight, *Baillieres Best Practice Research Clinical Endocrinology and Metabolism* 1999; (1): 109–120.
- Ayyad C & Anderson T, Long term efficacy of dietary treatment of obesity: a systematic review of studies published between 1931 and 1999, *Obesity Reviews* 2000; 1: 113-9.
- Brownell KD, *The Learn Programme for Weight Control*, Dallas: American Health Publishing Co.,1997.
- British Heart Foundation National Centre 'physical activity+health', Physical Activity Toolkit, BHF, 2001.
- Consumers' Association, *Which?*, May 2001, Diets: How the top selling diets measure up.
- Department of Health, *Nutritional Aspects of Cardiovascular disease*, Report of the Committee of

Medical Aspects of Food Policy (COMA). Report No. 46, London: HMSO, 1994.

▓ Department of Health, *Dietary Reference Values for Food Energy and Nutrients for the United Kingdom*. COMA Report No. 41, London: HMSO, 1991.

▓ Flechtner-Mors M et al., Metabolic and Weight-Loss Effects of a Long-Term Dietary Intervention in Obese Patients. Four-Year Results. *Obesity Research* 2000; 8: 399–402.

▓ Food Standards Agency, *The Balance of Good Health. Information for educators and communicators*, FSA, 2001.

▓ Freedman MR et al., Popular diets: a scientific review, *Obesity Research* 2001 Mar; 9 Suppl 1:1S–40S.

▓ Glenny A, O'Meara S, Melville A et al., A systematic review of the interventions for the prevention and treatment of obesity and the maintenance of weight loss, *International Journal of Obesity and Related Metabolic Disorders* 1997; 21: 9, 715–37.

▓ Golay A et al., Similar weight loss with low-energy food combining or balanced diets, *International Journal of Obesity & Related Metabolic Disorders* 2000; 24 (4): 492–6.

▓ Health Development Agency, Reducing Overweight and Obesity, in *Coronary Heart Disease: guidance for implementing the preventive aspects of the National Service Framework*, 2001.

▓ Hunt P & Hillsdon M, *Changing Eating and Exercise Behaviour. A Handbook for Professionals*, Oxford: Blackwell Science, 1996.

▓ Jebb AS & Goldberg GR, Efficacy of very low energy diets and meal replacements in the treatment of obesity, *Journal of Human Nutrition and Dietetics* 1998; 11: 219–25.

▓ Kayman S et al. Maintenance and relapse after weight loss in women: behavioral aspects. *American Journal of Clinical Nutrition* 1990; 52; 800-8-7.

▓ Klem ML etal. A descriptive study of individuals successful at long-term maintenance of substantial weight loss. *American Journal of Clinical Nutrition* 1997; 66(2): 239-46.

▓ Liu S et al., Whole-grain consumption and risk of coronary heart disease: results from the Nurses' Health Study, *American Journal of Clinical Nutrition* 1999; 70 (3): 412–9.

▓ Ludwig DS, The glycemic index: physiological mechanisms relating to obesity, diabetes, and cardiovascular disease, *Journal of the American Medical Association* 2002; 287 (18): 2414–23.

▓ National Institutes of Health, National Heart, Lung and Blood Institute, Clinical guidelines on the identification, evaluation and treatment of overweight and obesity in adults: the evidence report, 1999. www.nhlbi.nih.gov/health/prof/heart/index.htm#obesity

▓ Royal College of Physicians, *Overweight and Obese Patients: Principles of Management with Particular Reference to the Use of Drugs*, London: RCP, 1997.

▓ Sachiko T et al., AHA Scientific Advisory, Dietary protein and weight reduction, *Circulation* 2001; 104: 1869.

▓ Scottish Intercollegiate Guidelines Network, *Obesity in Scotland. Integrating Prevention with Weight Management*. Pilot Edition. Edinburgh: SIGN, 1996.

▓ Summerbell CD et al., Randomised controlled trial of novel, simple, and well-supervised weight reducing diets in outpatients, *British Medical Journal* 1998; 317: 1487–9.

▓ Treasure J & Schmidt U, Getting better bit(e) by bit(e). A survival kit for sufferers of bulimia nervosa and binge eating disorders. Clinician's Guide. London: Psychology Press, 1997.

▓ USDA Report on Popular Weight Loss Diets, Executive Summary, January 2001.

▓ Wardle J et al., *Shape-Up. A Lifestyle Programme to Manage your Weight*. London: Weight Concern, 2001. www.shape-up.org

▓ Wardle J & Rapoport L, Cognitive-Behavioural Treatment of Obesity, in P Kopelman & M Stock (eds), *Clincial Obesity*, London: Blackwell, 1998

INDEX